Negative Schizophrenic Symptoms: Pathophysiology and Clinical Implications

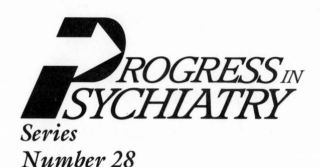

Series
Number 28

David Spiegel, M.D.,
Series Editor

Negative Schizophrenic Symptoms: Pathophysiology and Clinical Implications

Edited by
John F. Greden, M.D.
Rajiv Tandon, M.D.

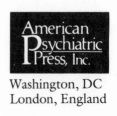

Washington, DC
London, England

Note: The authors have worked to ensure that all information in this book concerning drug dosages, schedules, and routes of administration is accurate as of the time of publication and consistent with standards set by the U.S. Food and Drug Administration and the general medical community. As medical research and practice advance, however, therapeutic standards may change. For this reason and because human and mechanical errors sometimes occur, we recommend that readers follow the advice of a physician who is directly involved in their care or the care of a member of their family.

Books published by the American Psychiatric Press, Inc., represent the views and opinions of the individual authors and do not necessarily represent the policies and opinions of the Press or the American Psychiatric Association.

Copyright © 1991 American Psychiatric Press, Inc.
ALL RIGHTS RESERVED
Manufactured in the United States of America
First Printing   93 92 91 90 4 3 2 1

American Psychiatric Press, Inc.
1400 K Street, N.W., Washington, DC 20005

The paper used in this publication meets the minimum requirements of the American National Standard for Information Sciences—Permanence of Paper for Printed Library Materials, ANSI Z39.48-1984.   ∞

Library of Congress Cataloging-in-Publication Data

Negative schizophrenic symptoms: pathophysiology and clinical implications/edited by John F. Greden, Rajiv Tandon.—1st ed.
        p.   cm. — (Progress in psychiatry; no. 28)
    Includes bibliographical references.
    ISBN 0-88048-192-7 (alk. paper)
    1. Schizophrenia—Pathophysiology. I. Greden, John F.,
1942–II. Tandon, Rajiv, 1956–   . III. Series.
    [DNLM: 1. Schizophrenia—physiopathology.
2. Schizophrenia—therapy. 3. Schizophrenic Psychology.
WM 203 N384]
RC514.N414   1990
616.89'82—dc20
DNLM/DLC   90-535
for Library of Congress   CIP

British Cataloguing in Publication Data

A CIP record is available from the British Library.

To Renee and Nammi,
Daniel, Sarah, Leigh, Neeraj, and Anisha,
for their love and patience

And to those who have assisted
us in studying schizophrenia by
providing financial support. We especially
acknowledge the National Alliance for
Research in Schizophrenia and Affective
Disorders (NARSAD), the Scottish Rite
Schizophrenia Program, and the
Theophile Raphael Fund

Contents

Treatment

Contributors

Nancy C. Andreasen, M.D., Ph.D.
Professor of Psychiatry, The University of Iowa College of Medicine, Iowa City, Iowa

Karen Faith Berman, M.D.
Clinical Brain Disorders Branch, Intramural Research Program, National Institute of Mental Health, Bethesda, Maryland; Neuroscience Center at Saint Elizabeths, Washington, DC

J. Brar, M.B.B.S.
Research Assistant, Department of Psychiatry, Western Psychiatric Institute and Clinic, University of Pittsburgh, Pittsburgh, Pennsylvania

Robert W. Buchanan, M.D.
Research Assistant Professor, Maryland Psychiatric Research Center, Department of Psychiatry, University of Maryland, Baltimore, Maryland.

William T. Carpenter, Jr., M.D.
Director, Maryland Psychiatric Research Center, Department of Psychiatry, University of Maryland School of Medicine, Baltimore, Maryland

Jeffrey A. Coffman, M.D.
Assistant Professor, Schizophrenia Research Program, Department of Psychiatry, The Ohio State University College of Medicine, Columbus, Ohio

Robert R. Conley, M.D.
Attending Psychiatrist, Spring Grove Hospital Center; Assistant Professor, University of Maryland School of Medicine, Baltimore, Maryland

Timothy J. Crow, M.B., F.R.C.P., Ph.D.
Head, Division of Psychiatry; Deputy Director, Clinical Research Centre, Northwick Park Hospital, Harrow, United Kingdom

John F. Dequardo, M.D.
Fellow, Schizophrenia Program, Chief Resident, Department of Psychiatry, University of Michigan Medical Center, Ann Arbor, Michigan

Alice Foerster, M.B., M.R.C.P.
Genetics Section, Institute of Psychiatry, De Crespigny Park,
London, United Kingdom

John F. Greden, M.D.
Professor and Chairman, Department of Psychiatry, and Research
Scientist, Mental Health Research Institute, University of Michigan,
Ann Arbor, Michigan

Stanley R. Kay, Ph.D.
Chief of Schizophrenia Research, Department of Psychiatry
(Psychology), Albert Einstein College of Medicine/Montefiore
Medical Center, and Director of Psychological Research, Bronx
Psychiatric Center, Bronx, New York

Matcheri S. Keshavan, M.D.
Medical Director, Inpatient Schizophrenia Module, Western
Psychiatric Institute and Clinic; Assistant Professor, Department of
Psychiatry, University of Pittsburgh, Pittsburgh, Pennsylvania

Brian Kirkpatrick, M.D.
Research Assistant Professor, Maryland Psychiatric Research Center,
Department of Psychiatry, University of Maryland School of
Medicine, Baltimore, Maryland

Shon W. Lewis, M.B., M.R.C.P.
Senior Lecturer, Department of Psychiatry, Charing Cross Hospital,
Fulham Palace Road, London, United Kingdom

Cheryl Mazzara, M.D.
Resident, Department of Psychiatry, University of Michigan Medical
Center, Ann Arbor, Michigan

Herbert Y. Meltzer, M.D.
Douglas D. Bond Professor of Psychiatry, Case Western Reserve
University School of Medicine, Cleveland, Ohio

Sukdeb Mukherjee, M.D.
Associate Professor of Clinical Psychiatry, Columbia University
College of Physicians and Surgeons; and Chief, Department of
Clinical Neuropsychiatry, New York State Psychiatric Institute, New
York, New York

Robin M. Murray, M.B., F.R.C.P.
Dean, Institute of Psychiatry, De Crespigny Park, London, United
Kingdom

Henry A. Nasrallah, M.D.
Chairman, Department of Psychiatry, The Ohio State University
College of Medicine, Columbus, Ohio

Thomas Neylan, M.D.
Assistant Professor, Western Psychiatric Institute and Clinic,
University of Pittsburgh Medical School; Highland Drive VA Medical
Center, Pittsburgh, Pennsylvania

Stephen C. Olson, M.D.
Assistant Professor, Schizophrenia Research Program, Department of
Psychiatry, The Ohio State University College of Medicine,
Columbus, Ohio

Jeffrey L. Peters, M.D.
Assistant Professor, Western Psychiatric Institute and Clinic,
University of Pittsburgh Medical School; Highland Drive VA Medical
Center, Pittsburgh, Pennsylvania

Michael F. Pogue-Geile, Ph.D.
Assistant Professor of Psychiatry, Western Psychiatric Institute and
Clinic, Departments of Psychology and Psychiatry, University of
Pittsburgh, Pittsburgh, Pennsylvania

Ravinder Reddy, M.D.
Van Ameringen Investigator in Schizophrenia Research, Department
of Psychiatry, Columbia University College of Physicians and
Surgeons, New York, New York

David B. Schnur, M.D.
Assistant Clinical Professor of Psychiatry, Columbia University
College of Physicians and Surgeons, New York; and Clinical Director,
Special Treatment Unit, Creedmoor Psychiatric Center, Queens
Village, New York

Steven B. Schwarzkopf, M.D.
Assistant Professor, Schizophrenia Research Program, Department of
Psychiatry, The Ohio State University College of Medicine,
Columbus, Ohio

David Shaw, Ph.D.
Assistant Professor, Western Psychiatric Institute and Clinic,
University of Pittsburgh Medical School; Highland Drive VA Medical
Center, Pittsburgh, Pennsylvania

Kenneth R. Silk, M.D.
Associate Director, Schizophrenia Program, Clinical Assistant
Professor, Department of Psychiatry, University of Michigan, Ann
Arbor, Michigan

Rajiv Tandon, M.D.
Director, Schizophrenia Program, Assistant Professor, Department of
Psychiatry, University of Michigan, Ann Arbor, Michigan

Daniel P. van Kammen, M.D., Ph.D.
Chief of Staff and Professor of Psychiatry, Highland Drive VA
Medical Center; Professor, Western Psychiatric Institute and Clinic,
University of Pittsburgh Medical School, Pittsburgh, Pennsylvania

Welmoet B. van Kammen, Ph.D.
Associate Professor, Western Psychiatric Institute and Clinic,
University of Pittsburgh Medical School; Highland Drive VA Medical
Center, Pittsburgh, Pennsylvania

Daniel R. Weinberger, M.D.
Chief, Clinical Brain Disorders Branch, Intramural Research
Program, National Institute of Mental Health, Bethesda, Maryland;
Neuroscience Center at Saint Elizabeths, Washington, DC

Jeffrey Yao, Ph.D.
Assistant Professor, Western Psychiatric Institute and Clinic,
University of Pittsburgh Medical School; Highland Drive VA Medical
Center, Pittsburgh, Pennsylvania

Introduction to the
Progress in Psychiatry *Series*

The *Progress in Psychiatry* Series is designed to capture in print the excitement that comes from assembling a diverse group of experts from various locations to examine in detail the newest information about a developing aspect of psychiatry. This series emerged as a collaboration between the American Psychiatric Association's (APA) Scientific Program Committee and the American Psychiatric Press, Inc. Great interest is generated by a number of the symposia presented each year at the APA Annual Meeting, and we realized that much of the information presented there, carefully assembled by people who are deeply immersed in a given area, would unfortunately not appear together in print. The symposia sessions at the Annual Meetings provide an unusual opportunity for experts who otherwise might not meet on the same platform to share their diverse viewpoints for a period of 3 hours. Some new themes are repeatedly reinforced and gain credence, while in other instances disagreements emerge, enabling the audience and now the reader to reach informed decisions about new directions in the field. The *Progress in Psychiatry* Series allows us to publish and capture some of the best of the symposia and thus provide an in-depth treatment of specific areas that might not otherwise be presented in broader review formats.

Psychiatry is by nature an interface discipline, combining the study of mind and brain, of individual and social environments, of the humane and the scientific. Therefore, progress in the field is rarely linear—it often comes from unexpected sources. Further, new developments emerge from an array of viewpoints that do not necessarily provide immediate agreement but rather expert examination of the issues. We intend to present innovative ideas and data that will enable you, the reader, to participate in this process.

We believe the *Progress in Psychiatry* Series will provide you with an opportunity to review timely new information in specific fields of interest as they are developing. We hope you find that the excitement of the presentations is captured in the written word and that this book proves to be informative and enjoyable reading.

David Spiegel, M.D.
Series Editor
Progress in Psychiatry Series

Progress in Psychiatry *Series Titles*

Foreword

As this volume amply attests, the past decade has been characterized by an exuberant profusion of studies concerning the "negative" symptoms of schizophrenia. Much of the credit for rekindling interest in this topic goes to Tim Crow, whose views are represented in a chapter in this book, and who introduced a creative approach to the problem of reducing heterogeneity in the study of schizophrenia. Although there are differences in the language used to refer to the concept—negative symptoms, defect state, Type II syndrome, fundamental symptoms, deficit symptoms, or deficit state—there is a clear consensus about its importance. A return to an interest in negative symptoms is quite simply a return to the concepts of Kraepelin and Bleuler, founding fathers of the concept of "dementia praecox or the group of schizophrenias." Others in British and American psychiatry, such as Wing, Carpenter, or Strauss, have made important "historical" contributions as well, and continue to make ongoing contributions.

This return to an interest in the most fundamental symptoms of psychosis is not without problems, as this volume also amply attests. The profusion of interest has led to a profusion of competing concepts, competing definitions, competing rating scales, and competing models. Science differs from industry in that only a modest amount of competition is useful, and after a certain point a babble of concepts and terms is likely to lead to confusion rather than consensus. Through their thoughtful introduction and conclusion, Drs. Greden and Tandon have made a heroic effort to summarize the ways in which a useful consensus and integration may be achieved.

Because I was unable to contribute a chapter to the volume, I was asked to write a foreword instead to summarize my own insights and reflections. Although there is little to add to the rich abundance that has already been presented in this volume, a few points may bear reemphasis.

First, the disease that we refer to as schizophrenia is probably heterogeneous. Its phenomenologic heterogeneity is evident, and it is probably heterogeneous in its pathophysiology and etiology as well. This heterogeneity tends to blur the focus of all our studies, whether they be of clinical presentation, course, outcome, response to treatment, neurochemistry, neurophysiology, genetics, or the role of environmental factors. Although the distinction between positive (florid, Type I) schizophrenia and negative (deficit, Type II) schizophrenia offered a hope that this schema might reduce heterogeneity, it now seems clear that this dichotomization is only a heuristic oversimplification. Unfortunately, we still do not know how to reduce heterogeneity and identify discrete subtypes. Nevertheless, there are some long-term strategies that may help us gain leverage on the problem of schizophrenia and its related psychoses.

We should avoid premature closure. We do not know the true boundaries of the concept of schizophrenia, nor can we identify any single pathognomonic symptom. In such a situation, we investigators would do best to sample broadly from the schizophrenia spectrum, including patients with "core" schizophrenia as well as the syndromes we refer to as schizoaffective disorder, schizophreniform disorder, schizotypal disorder, simple schizophrenia, and delusional disorder. Quite possibly, at least with some patients, what is now called "mood incongruent psychosis" may also fall within the schizophrenia spectrum. Sampling should also be broad with respect to symptoms. Clinical assessment batteries should be as comprehensive as possible, and they should definitely not be limited to approaches that use only symptoms included in diagnostic criteria sets such as DSM-III or DSM-III-R. (This broader approach is exemplified in the structured interview that we have been developing for the past 5 years, the Comprehensive Assessment of Symptoms and History, or CASH).

The study of a broad variety of clinical signs and symptoms must be complemented with the study of a broad array of potentially informative biological measures. We should be well past the period of the "single illness—single marker" mentality. Instead, our thinking must be dimensional and must be firmly rooted in both clinical and basic neuroscience. Instead of asking, "Is there a biological marker for schizophrenia?" or even "Has the concept of schizophrenia been validated by studies of genetics or response to treatment?" we should be asking, "How are the symptoms that we observe in psychotic spectrum conditions mediated through neural mechanisms that occur interactively in the structural and biochemical circuits of the human brain as it develops from birth to old age?"

The requirements of so much breadth present an obvious challenge. Large samples are needed, and the host of variables produced are likely to be difficult to analyze statistically. Apart from the usual nostrum of clearly formulating a priori hypotheses to avoid the risk of Type I error in the presence of so much abundance, what else can one do? One useful strategy that has emerged during the past few years is the focus on highly informative populations. These include prospective longitudinal studies of first-episode patients, the study of monozygotic and dizygotic twins, the study of multiplex families, and the evaluation of patients who are homogeneous with respect to some important phenomenological characteristic (e.g., experiencing a clear "defect state"). To the largest extent possible, investigators should try to use similar instruments, assays, measurement techniques, and methods of assessment. Cross-center collaboration and standardization is likely to be more fruitful in the long run than cross-center competition and proliferation of methods, since this approach will clarify issues of nonreplicability.

The resurgence of interest in negative symptoms has restored a balance to descriptive psychopathology that was badly needed. We now recognize that psychosis is not defined by simple pathognomonic symptoms such as first-rank symptoms of Schneider, nor even by such objective all-or-none phenomena as delusions and hallucinations. We also recognize that we are not likely to understand the neurobiology of schizophrenia by examining a single neurotransmitter such as dopamine or a single etiologic mechanism such as autosomal dominant genetic transmission. This growth and maturity during the past decade should provide a firm foundation for the coming one, aptly identified as the Decade of the Brain and of the Schizophrenia Initiative. By the year 2000 we may not have discovered the cause of schizophrenia, but we will certainly know much more.

Nancy C. Andreasen, M.D., Ph.D.

Introduction

S ince Emil Kraepelin (1919) and Eugen Bleuler (1950) con-
solidated the concepts of dementia praecox and schizophrenia
almost a century ago, the heterogeneity of the disorder has been
recognized as a problem. Clinicians and investigators have struggled
to identify the syndrome's core in terms of its symptomatology,
genetic liability, association with various neurobiologic abnormalities,
treatment response, longitudinal course, and outcome. Two general
strategies have been employed to delineate etiologically distinct
categories of schizophrenic illness. One was based on a descriptive
approach (phenomenology, longitudinal course, and outcome) and
the other (more recent) relied on underlying neurobiologic correlates.
Unfortunately, the various approaches employed so far have failed to
forge a consensus.

Over the past decade, there has been increasing emphasis on
dichotomization of schizophrenic illness based on the positive-negative symptom distinction. This method combines the descriptive and
neurobiologic strategies and attempts to bring together data from
clinical phenomenology, genetic liability, premorbid development,
biological correlates, treatment response, longitudinal course, and
outcome.

"Negative" symptoms such as apathy, amotivation, anhedonia,
avolition, blunted affect, emotional withdrawal, and impoverished
speech and thinking have been considered by many to be essential
features of schizophrenic illness. Early theoreticians, including
Kraepelin and Bleuler, considered them to represent "fundamental"
or "core" psychopathologies. Over the years, however, their importance was progressively downplayed. Increasing emphasis was placed
on positive symptoms such as delusions and hallucinations, as
epitomized by the publication and almost universal acceptance of
Schneider's (1959) checklist of "first-rank" schizophrenic symptoms,
which consisted exclusively of positive symptoms. Factors contributing to this trend included

1. The difficulty in reliably defining and documenting negative symptoms, in contrast to positive symptoms, which could be more reliably defined and measured
2. The more florid expression of positive symptoms
3. The revolution in treatment of schizophrenia brought about by the introduction of neuroleptics, which produce the most dramatic improvement in positive symptoms. (Although negative symptoms also improve with neuroleptic treatment, this effect is less discernible, and certainly less dramatic.)

Despite widespread acceptance of Schneider's checklist, however, the positive symptoms were unable to provide an adequate characterization of schizophrenia. In fact, these were found to correlate poorly with chronicity and deterioration, considered central to traditional definitions of schizophrenia. Furthermore, the almost universal presence and relative persistence of negative symptomatology, combined with the fact that they constitute the most debilitating and refractory aspect of schizophrenic psychopathology, made them difficult to ignore.

Strauss et al. (1974) reintroduced the positive-negative symptom distinction to the study of schizophrenia. Further impetus for recent empirical work was provided by Crow (1980a) and Andreasen (1982), both of whom explored the utility of schizophrenic subtypes based on the positive-negative symptom distinction. In contrast to positive symptoms, negative symptoms were generally found to be more chronic and persistent, less responsive to neuroleptic treatment, associated with inadequate premorbid adjustment and poor social functioning, accompanied by a greater probability of cognitive impairment and computed tomography evidence of cerebral atrophy, and associated with poor outcome. Attempts to understand these apparently different profiles led to the suggestion that although positive symptoms were related to dopaminergic hyperactivity, negative symptoms might be linked to other brain abnormalities.

During the past 10 years, research on negative symptoms has mushroomed. There have been more than 1,000 relevant publications, and at least three major journals have devoted special issues to the topic (*Schizophrenia Bulletin* Vol. 11, No. 3, 1985; *International Journal of Mental Health*, Vol. 16, No 4, 1988; *British Journal of Psychiatry*, Special issue, 1989). Researchers have generated enormous amounts of data on various aspects of negative symptomatology and have compared these data with positive symptoms on many dimensions. These studies generally have provided support for the utility of the positive-negative distinction. These developments attest to the great promise and growing impact of the negative-symptom syndrome as an organizing construct in schizophrenia.

As literature in this field grew, however, some important problems emerged. Conceptual and methodological limitations became apparent. A number of conflicting and contradictory findings were noted. Several competing definitions of the negative-symptom concept emerged. The terminology became confusing, and vastly different terms (with vastly different implications)—such as *negative, deficit, defect, Type II,* and *residual*—are now being used interchangeably. More than a dozen rating scales, each with its own conceptual bias and construct limitations, are being utilized to measure and define this concept. The issue of whether a particular rating instrument matches the theoretical bias of the rater and can serve the purpose of negative-symptom assessment in a given study has received little attention. Distinctions between primary and secondary negative symptoms have generally not been made, and the longitudinal perspective has often been ignored. To add to this confusion, various structural, biochemical, developmental, etiologic, and pathophysiologic mechanisms have been implicated to explain negative symptomatology. All of these problems lead to difficulties in generalizing from one study to another.

In this volume, we present current information on negative symptoms; discuss the validity of various competing concepts; review current biochemical, structural, and developmental theories to explain negative symptoms; outline pharmacologic and other treatment approaches; and delineate promising areas for future research. In the first section—"Concept and Phenomenology"—the concepts and clinical features of the negative-symptom syndrome are discussed. Drs. Carpenter, Buchanan, and Kirkpatrick review the historical development of the concept and discuss the validity of competing definitions. Dr. Kay discusses the validity of various definitions of the negative-symptom construct with specific reference to the short- and long-term longitudinal course of negative symptoms in schizophrenia. The concepts of syndrome and subtype are central to research on negative symptoms, and Drs. Pogue-Geile and Keshavan discuss the empirical evidence with regard to the syndrome and subtype status of negative symptoms in schizophrenia. Drs. Silk and Tandon discuss the theoretical bias, content, and administration of the various rating scales used to assess negative symptoms.

In the next section—"Biochemical Hypotheses"—the contributors review various biochemical hypotheses formulated to explain negative symptoms. Drs. Berman and Weinberger present evidence that suggests a relative deficiency of dopamine in certain crucial brain areas and an imbalance among the various components of the dopamine system as key pathogenic features of negative symptoms. Drs. Tandon and Greden review evidence implicating muscarinic cholinergic hyperactivity in the production of negative symptoms and present a model of cholinergic-dopaminergic interactions in the context of the longitudinal course of schizophrenia. Drs. van Kammen, Peters, Yao, van Kammen, Neylan, and Shaw present data implicating noradrenergic dysregulation in the production of negative symptoms, suggesting that whereas increased noradrenergic activity may be involved in the production of both positive and negative symptoms in the psychotic phase of schizophrenia, decreased noradrenergic activity may contribute to "deficit" symptoms in the chronic, residual phase of the illness. Drs. Keshavan, Mazzara, Brar, and Dequardo review data from the psychoneuroendocrine literature, linking these to various biochemical theories of negative symptoms in schizophrenia.

In the third section of the book—"Structural and Developmental Theories"—prevailing structural, developmental, and genetic theories of negative schizophrenic symptoms are discussed. Drs. Olson, Nasrallah, Coffman, and Schwarzkopf review data on various structural abnormalities in schizophrenia as they pertain to the presence of the negative syndrome. Dr. Crow summarizes his present understanding of the negative syndrome and views the structural changes associated with negative symptoms in the context of a developmental perspective. Drs. Mukherjee, Reddy, and Schnur examine the relationship between aspects of premorbid functioning and negative symptoms in schizophrenic patients, linking different components of the negative syndrome to different stages of development. Drs. Foerster, Lewis, and Murray examine the interactive roles of genetic and environmental factors in the production of positive and negative syndromes in schizophrenia.

The fourth section of this book—Treatment—addresses treatment approaches to negative symptoms. Drs. Carpenter and Conley discuss the overall approach to the management of negative symptoms, highlight the need to distinguish primary from secondary negative symptoms, and outline several behavioral and rehabilitation strategies. Dr. Meltzer discusses pharmacologic approaches to the treatment of negative symptoms.

In the final chapter of the book, Drs. Tandon and Greden inquire as to how the various concepts and pathophysiologic theories of the negative-symptom construct might be integrated.

Renewed interest in negative symptoms is encouraging. Although dichotomizations, if rigidly and ideologically applied, often impede the progress of science, the heuristic dichotomization of schizophrenic symptoms as positive and negative has explained some important features of the illness and promises to aid us in understanding further the heterogeneity of schizophrenia. We recognize that although we remain at an early stage of understanding, data are rapidly accumulating to guide our future conceptualizations, evaluations, and treatments. We hope that this volume, by clarifying our current state of knowledge, will contribute to the growing momentum and lead to more efficacious treatment in this critical area.

John F. Greden, M.D.
Rajiv Tandon, M.D.

Concept and Phenomenology

Chapter 1

The Concept of the Negative Symptoms of Schizophrenia

William T. Carpenter, Jr., M.D.
Robert W. Buchanan, M.D.
Brian Kirkpatrick, M.D.

Chapter 1

The Concept of the Negative Symptoms of Schizophrenia

An understanding of negative symptoms is of paramount importance, both to the clinician responsible for the care of the schizophrenic patient and to the investigator attempting to formulate explanatory hypotheses concerning the cause and pathophysiology of schizophrenia. This profound erosion of experience and behavior is one of the most devastating effects of the illness process. Often beginning early in life and lasting into old age, this group of impairments accounts for much of the enormous personal and financial burden associated with schizophrenia. Furthermore, the negative symptom component may best distinguish one of the most prevalent chronic forms of schizophrenia. Despite the centrality of negative symptoms in the psychopathology of schizophrenia, however, it is only recently that a sharp focus on this concept has led to hypotheses and data of specific relevance to this core phenomenon. Yet even as progress unfolds, the field is encumbered with competing concepts and assessment approaches, and a myriad of confounding issues that reduce the opportunity for studying negative symptoms.

In this chapter, we will review the development of the negative symptom concept, propose an approach to the core psychopathology construct, and present data that provide tentative support for its validity. We hope that this conceptualization will be of value in directing future research.

HISTORICAL OVERVIEW

Strauss et al. (1974) reintroduced the negative symptom terminology

---

Supported in part by NIMH grants MH-40279, MH-35996, MH-09044; a grant from the Scottish Rite Schizophrenia Research Program, Northern Masonic Jurisdiction; and the National Alliance for Research in Schizophrenia and Affective Disorders (NARSAD) Fellowship Extension Award (R.W.B.).

to the area of schizophrenia research, citing the advantages of distinguishing among three general types of psychopathologic manifestations: positive symptoms, negative symptoms, and disorders of relating. Although excellent descriptions dating back to Kraepelin (1919) and Bleuler (1950) were available, John Hughlings Jackson's (1875, 1889) terminology was selected because of its descriptive value. Jackson described positive symptoms as the excesses in normal brain processes; negative symptoms were the diminution or negation of normal processes. Jackson's concept of the hierarchical organization of the brain, however, with its implication that negative symptoms result from tissue destruction and positive symptoms are disinhibiting consequences of this tissue destruction, was not accepted. Rather, positive symptoms such as hallucinations and delusions were differentiated from negative symptoms such as restricted affect and anergia solely at the descriptive level. Both were viewed as primary components of schizophrenia.

Berrios (1985) provided an informative historical overview of the development of the positive and negative symptom concepts. He traced the concept to an 1857 paper in which John Russell Reynolds stated "Many of the symptoms of disease are merely modified vital actions . . . some symptoms are negative, i.e., they consist in the negation of vital properties . . . other symptoms are positive, i.e., they consist in the excess of alteration of vital properties."

In this view, positive and negative symptoms are the results of the fluctuation of vital energy; they were not placed in a hierarchy where one was primary and the other secondary. According to Berrios, de Clerambault introduced the positive and negative concept directly into psychiatry, describing positive symptoms as phenomena such as hallucinations and delusions, and negative symptoms as "inhibitory" phenomena such as thought withdrawal, perplexity, and attentional impairment. Here, too, no direct or hierarchical relationship is assumed between positive and negative symptoms.

Today, most workers accept positive and negative at the descriptive level, but there is no unanimity as to whether these two symptom domains are directly related, inversely related, or independent processes. Some workers postulate different etiology and pathogenesis, whereas others suggest unifying theoretical constructs (Schizophrenia Bulletin 1985).

Kraepelin (1919) provided the most compelling framework for distinguishing positive and negative symptoms. He referred to the two groups of maladies of dementia praecox:

> Now if we make a general survey of the psychic clinical picture of

dementia praecox . . . there are apparently two principal groups of disorders which characterize the malady. On the one hand we observe a weakening of those emotional activities which permanently form the mainsprings of volition. . . . The result of this part of the morbid process is emotional dullness, failure of mental activities, loss of mastery over volition, of endeavor, and of ability for independent action. The essence of personality is thereby destroyed, the best and most precious part of its being, as Griesinger once expressed it, torn from her. With the annihilation of personal will, the possibility of further development is lost, which is dependent wholly on the activity of volition. (pp. 74–75)

Bleuler (1950) also described psychopathology relevant to these two domains, although he suggested dissociative phenomena were primary and many other pathologic manifestations were secondary. Bleuler's hierarchical argument, however, does not fit neatly into the positive-negative dichotomy.

Strauss et al. (1974) provided the following descriptive proposals for positive and negative symptoms:

Data suggest the utility of postulating that three major types of processes underlie schizophrenic symptoms and signs. These three hypothetical processes can be arrived at by grouping the six kinds of symptoms into three categories: positive symptoms, negative symptoms, and disorders in relating. . . . We use these terms here primarily descriptively without necessarily implying Jackson's theoretical conceptions, but find the terms useful because symptoms within each of the groups appear to have some important basic similarities in their relationship to antecedents and outcome. In this way, the concepts of positive and negative symptoms may help shed light on the basic pathological processes involved in schizophrenia. As Jackson described them, positive symptoms are those that have the appearance of being active processes—for example, delusions, hallucinations, and catatonic motor phenomena. In a discussion of this group of symptoms, Snezhnevsky considers them similar also because of their relative flexibility. Negative symptoms, on the other hand, involve primarily absence of normal functions. In schizophrenia, negative symptoms include such phenomena as blunting of affect, apathy, and certain kinds of formal thought disorder, such as blocking. Snezhnevsky describes the inflexibility of this group of symptoms. (p. 65)

Symptoms manifest in the interpersonal sphere may represent a different domain, but it is also evident that both positive and negative symptoms can underlie pathologic manifestations in this sphere.

Three general approaches have been taken to this area. In conceptualizing Type I and Type II schizophrenia, Crow (1985) attempted to subdivide the syndrome according to multiple criteria, with the greatest emphasis being placed on the presence or absence of negative symptoms. Crow's criteria are based on items from the Manchester

Scale (Krawiecka et al. 1977), with poverty of speech and restricted affect defining the presence of the negative symptom syndrome (Type II). The prominence of psychotic symptoms, however, is apparently also part of these criteria, specifically in the definition of Type I schizophrenia (Crow 1985). This construct has led to a series of studies, many of which provide supporting and validating data, demonstrating the importance of subdividing a heterogeneous clinical syndrome such as schizophrenia. A problem with this approach with respect to its heuristic value for research, however, is the delineation of two hypothesized disease entities by multiple criteria. Consequently, when differences are found, it cannot always be ascertained whether the presence of the negative symptom domain was the crucial contributing factor. Generally, multiple and diverse criteria are optimal for defining disease entities, but not for defining specific pathologic phenomena.

A second approach, put forward by Andreasen and Olsen (1982), conceptualizes positive and negative symptoms as different ends of the same continuum and describes patients as either predominantly positive or predominantly negative. This approach has several problems at the level of categorical assignment. In the first place, positive symptoms tend to fluctuate, so how "positive" a patient may be is highly dependent on time of assessment. This stricture is also true of transitory forms of negative symptoms. Second, most studies fail to support the hypothesis of an inverse relationship between positive and negative symptoms (Lewine et al. 1983; Pogue-Geile and Harrow 1984; Walker et al. 1988). There are reports of a negative correlation, but there is also the possibility that such a correlation is dependent on the phase of illness. The more chronic or "burned out" cases will fall into the negative group; the same patients at earlier phases of illness might have been designated as primarily positive. Although this approach may be satisfactory for current state description, it does not provide a basis for etiologic exploration. There is also the commonplace problem of observation of the simultaneous manifestation of severe positive and negative symptoms.

A third approach is based on domains of psychopathology, in which each domain is isolated for study in its own right and can provide a basis for subdividing the schizophrenia syndrome on that dimension alone (Carpenter and Buchanan 1989). With this approach, correlates can be directly related to the presence or absence of the negative symptom psychopathology per se. Preliminary results subdividing schizophrenia on the basis of a negative symptom domain are presented below.

PRESENT CONCEPTS

Central to the investigation of negative symptoms in schizophrenia is the question of which symptoms should be included. We will address this issue first, then discuss the primary-secondary distinction and the transitory-enduring distinction.

Most investigators have used the negative symptom concept to refer to the diminution or loss of normal functions, and a long list of candidate symptoms, selected from the affective, cognitive, and social spheres of behavior, has been generated (see Walker and Lewine 1988). There is some consensus that this list can be reduced to the following symptoms: blunted or restricted affect, poverty of speech, loss of drive, social and emotional withdrawal, anhedonia, apathy, poor grooming, motor retardation, and impaired social relationships (Andreasen 1982; Carpenter et al. 1985; Crow 1985; Iager et al. 1985; Kay et al. 1987b; Walker and Lewine 1988). This consensus is based, in part, on investigations that have brought into question the validity of including certain symptoms—for example, attentional impairment, inappropriate affect, and certain forms of thought disorder (loose associations and incoherent and irrelevant speech)—as negative symptoms (Andreasen and Olsen 1982; Bilder et al. 1985; Gibbons et al. 1985; Kay et al. 1987b; Pogue-Geile and Harrow 1985; Walker et al. 1988). We ourselves have reservations about poor grooming, motor retardation, and impaired social relationships.

Poor grooming and impaired social relationships are derivative symptoms and may well be secondary to psychosis per se. Motor retardation is a poor conceptual fit, and its frequent occurrence in major affective disorders lessens its interest as a possible core symptom of schizophrenia.

The "true" set of negative symptoms is not yet known, but the importance of these symptoms for scientific inquiry requires that we make our best "guess" as to which symptoms should be included for study. In the absence of a well-developed theoretical framework for selecting negative symptoms, we suggest that certain conceptual distinctions be made to derive from the list of putative symptoms the most conceptually valid set for investigation.

The first conceptual issue relates to the differentiation of primary from secondary or derivative negative symptoms. If negative symptoms are to be useful in the study of schizophrenia, they should be the direct manifestation of a specific pathophysiologic process in schizophrenia (Carpenter and Buchanan 1989; Carpenter et al. 1988). This statement need not imply that the pathologic process is unique to schizophrenia. Rather, the process is a core characteristic in schizophrenia that is relatively capable of differentiating between schizophrenia and other psychiatric syndromes. In discerning the presence of any putative negative symptoms, a careful differential diagnosis excluding neuroleptic effect, dysphoric mood, under-stimulating environment, and any other potential causative factor needs to be made (Carpenter et al. 1985, 1988). For example, failure to differentiate primary anhedonia from anhedonia secondary to depression would reduce the power of the negative symptom concept by confounding negative symptoms with affective symptomatology. A similar problem arises if, in the assessment of a negative symptom, a derivative behavioral manifestation of the negative symptom is assessed rather than the symptom itself. An example of this problem is equating social withdrawal with diminished social drive. A schizophrenic patient may be socially withdrawn because of a primary diminution of social drive, as a self-protective mechanism to reduce stimulation during psychosis, or as avoidance behavior based on paranoid ideation. Social withdrawal is, therefore, a poor proxy if diminished social drive is the psychopathology of interest.

A second conceptual issue is concerned with the differentiation of transitory state from enduring trait negative symptoms. Theoretically, primary negative symptoms may be either transitory or enduring. The difficulty arises in trying to make the primary-secondary distinction when the symptom manifestation is brief (Carpenter et al. 1985). The use of enduring negative symptoms would enhance the accuracy of the primary-secondary distinction and has a theoretical basis as well. It is, after all, these enduring manifestations that Kraepelin described and that are implied in most present-day investigations. The study of acute or transitory negative symptoms is needed but also requires the state-trait distinction.

These principles can be used to define putative subtypes based on the presence of primary negative symptoms of the enduring or transitory type. Common usage and historical precedent carry weight as to the choice of specific negative symptoms, but theory also provides guidance. We will outline two such possibilities.

One theoretical approach is based on an anatomic argument. Patients with known focal lesions have been reported to show impairments similar to those found in putative negative symptom subtypes. For instance, enduring poverty of speech, blunted affect, diminished social drive, and diminished sense of purpose have been noted in patients with lesions of the amygdala (Jacobson 1986; Scoville et al. 1953; Terzian and Ore 1955), and in some patients with focal prefrontal lesions (Ackerly and Benton 1947; Blumer and Benson 1975; Brickner 1934, 1936; Fuster 1980; Hebb 1945; Hecaen and

Albert 1975; Milner 1964; Nauta 1971; Penfield and Evans 1935). These neurologic data are limited; the studies have not focused on those impairments that resemble schizophrenia, and there are contradictions in the literature. Nonetheless, the resemblance to the negative symptoms of schizophrenia suggests that intensive study of such patients will help delineate a negative symptom subtype sharing this anatomic substrate.

Neuroethology provides a second theoretical approach. Bilateral lesions of the amygdala cause mammals to become social isolates who do not seek normal physical proximity to conspecifics or participate in social interactions such as grooming. This behavior is not based on active avoidance (Aggleton and Passingham 1981; Bunnell 1966; Bunnell et al. 1970; Chozick 1985; Dicks et al. 1969; Fonberg and Kostarczyk 1980; Jonason and Enloe 1971; Kling and Steklis 1976; Mass and Kling 1975; Myers and Swett 1970; Myers et al. 1973; Rosvold et al. 1954; Steklis et al. 1975; Zagrodzka et al. 1983). Such animals thus provide a model for diminished social drive. The same animals are able to display normal social communicative cues (vocalizations, facial expressions), but do so very rarely; thus such lesions may model blunted affect and poverty of speech (Kling 1972; Kling and Steklis 1976; Myers and Swett 1970; Ploog 1981). These impairments are not found after lesions in several other brain areas (Gray and McNaughton 1983; Jonason and Enloe 1971; Murphy et al. 1981; Myers et al. 1973; Poplawsky and Johnson 1973; Steklis et al. 1975). Single cell recordings have shown that there are cells in the amygdala, primarily in the basolateral area, that respond selectively to faces of members of the same species (Leonard et al. 1985). Schizophrenic patients have also been noted to have abnormalities in the visual processing of faces (Morrison et al. 1988). Thus the features of amygdalar lesions suggest that diminished social drive, blunted affect, and poverty of speech may have a common neural basis, and that this constellation of attributes may represent appropriate aspects of the definition of a negative symptom subtype.

These neurologic and neuroethological models must be viewed with caution. Even if there is substantial descriptive similarity between the models and a negative symptom subtype, the etiology of the relevant behaviors can differ in important ways from the disease process of schizophrenia. These models, however, deserve more consideration, as they suggest that damage to the putative neural circuit mediating social affiliation (Kling and Steklis 1976) may underlie the enduring negative symptoms of schizophrenia.

We have identified six negative symptoms (i.e., poverty of speech, diminished emotional range, blunted affect, diminished sense of purpose, curbing of interests, and diminished social drive) that we believe merit study, and we propose the use of the term *deficit* to refer to these symptoms when they are present in the primary, enduring form (Carpenter et al. 1988). Taken together, a deficit process can be defined that may reduce the heterogeneity of schizophrenia by subtyping patients into deficit and nondeficit cohorts. The reliability and validity of this approach will be discussed below.

DELINEATION OF A NEGATIVE SYMPTOM SUBTYPE: THE DEFICIT SYNDROME

Despite wide agreement on the importance of negative symptoms, they play a small part in "modern" criteria for schizophrenia. One rationale for emphasizing hallucinations and delusions in criteria for schizophrenia was the alleged poor reliability of negative symptoms. It has been shown, however, that good reliability can in fact be achieved in this area (Andreasen 1982; Heinrichs et al. 1984; Kay et al. 1987a). In the late 1960s, putative negative symptoms such as restricted affect and poor rapport were reliably observed in a multinational study and proved highly discriminating of a schizophrenic diagnosis (Carpenter et al. 1973; World Health Organization 1974).

Defining subtypes is a task different from that of describing the association between negative symptoms and other variables. The literature is replete with correlations, but usually not with emphasis on primary negative symptoms. These associations are reviewed in several chapters in this volume and are beyond the scope of this chapter. Andreasen (1985) also reviewed these data. We will not consider the positive versus negative dichotomy for four reasons. First, most studies fail to support the proposed inverse relationship (Cornblatt et al. 1985; Lewine 1985; Pogue-Geile and Harrow 1984; Walker et al. 1988). Second, positive symptoms are required for a diagnosis of schizophrenia. If ubiquitous, they can be only a dichotomizing tool as state phenomena (e.g., no positive symptoms today), lessening their value for studies of etiology and correlation with trait variables. Third, the positive versus negative distinction is often based on the SANS methodology (Andreasen 1982), which does not purport to distinguish primary from secondary or transient from enduring negative symptoms. Fourth, an excellent update on positive versus negative schizophrenia has been published (Andreasen 1990b). We will therefore focus primarily on the Type II and deficit forms of schizophrenia.

Little attention has been paid to the reliability of subtypes based on negative symptoms. To standardize the categorization of patients into deficit and nondeficit groups, the Schedule for the Deficit Syndrome

(SDS) was developed. The SDS, based in part on the Quality of Life Scale (Heinrichs et al. 1984), describes the features used to make the diagnosis, outlines a method of scoring, and provides instructions for assessing the patient.

To test the reliability of the SDS, two raters assessed 40 patients who met DSM-III (American Psychiatric Association 1980) criteria for schizophrenia. Patients were interviewed during clinical stability (i.e., between flagrant episodes of psychotic exacerbation). Information was also gathered from other sources to assess characteristics of usual functioning. Interrater reliability was good for the deficit-nondeficit categorization, individual deficit symptoms, and global severity. The kappa value for the simple global categorization (i.e., deficit versus nondeficit) was .73. The weighted kappa values for the six negative symptoms used to define the deficit syndrome were restricted affect, .74; diminished emotional range, .68; poverty of speech, .69; curbing of interests, .66; diminished sense of purpose, .69; and diminished social drive, .60. For global severity, the weighted kappa was .72. Parenthetically, discrepancies on categorization or global severity were easily resolved with discussion, suggesting consensus ratings would enhance validity.

Patients in the Chestnut Lodge long-term follow-up study also have been categorized into deficit and nondeficit groups with good reliability, using published criteria (Carpenter et al. 1988; Fenton and McGlashan, personal communications).

Are subtypes defined by negative symptoms valid and meaningful? Proposed negative symptom dichotomies are the Type I versus Type II schizophrenia of Crow (1985) and the deficit versus nondeficit schizophrenia of Carpenter et al. (1988).

Validity of the Type I–Type II Categorization

Crow (1985) used poverty of speech and blunted affect as the key symptoms for the definition of a negative symptom subtype because of his belief that these are the symptoms that are both primary and enduring. In a study of the efficacy of two isomers of flupentixol, these symptoms did not show a therapeutic response when compared with placebo (Johnstone et al. 1978a). These negative symptoms are reported to be associated with intellectual impairment and neurologic signs (Crow and Mitchell 1975; Crow and Stevens 1978; Owens and Johnstone 1980). Crow (1985) also argued that ventricular enlargement occurs most frequently in Type II patients and is due to an abnormality in the temporal lobe. In a recent study, patients with enlarged ventricles, consistent with Crow's hypothesis, were shown to be less responsive to treatment and amphetamine challenge (Pandurangi et al. 1989).

Other postmortem studies have more directly supported the validity of Type II schizophrenia. Type II patients were found to have less cholecystokinin immunoreactivity in the hippocampus and amygdala than did controls, whereas Type I patients did not differ from controls (Ferrier et al. 1983a; Roberts et al. 1983). Owen et al. (1987) also found an association between Type II clinical characteristics and a decrease in monoamine oxidase-B concentrations in frontal and temporal cortex, as well as amygdala, in comparison to Type I patients.

A neuroendocrinologic marker may also be associated with Type II schizophrenia. Schizophrenic patients exhibit an unusually high prevalence of both abnormally elevated and abnormally low growth hormone (GH) peaks following the administration of the dopaminergic agonist apomorphine. Several correlates have been proposed for the abnormally elevated peak (see Zemlan et al. 1986a for review). The blunted response, which has been found in patients never exposed to neuroleptics (Cleghorn et al. 1983a; Ferrier et al. 1984), occurs primarily in "chronic" patients (Ferrier et al. 1984; Meltzer et al. 1984; Pandey et al. 1977), but it may be a marker of a negative symptom subtype. Negative symptoms were associated with a blunted GH response in two studies (Ferrier et al. 1984; Tamminga et al. 1977), but were weakly associated with an enhanced GH response in another study (Meltzer et al. 1986). This discrepancy may be explained by population differences, as Meltzer et al. (1984) studied acutely relapsed patients, and such cohorts included many patients whose negative symptoms improve as their psychotic symptoms diminish (Goldberg 1985). In contrast, the other two teams studied very chronic groups.

Ferrier et al. (1984) also found negative symptoms correlated with a blunted GH response in a mixed group of chronic and acute schizophrenic patients; the patients in the chronic group had been drug-free for at least a year, and 5 of the 15 had never received neuroleptic treatment. This correlation was also statistically significant within the chronic group alone, after accounting for the effects of age, which correlates with duration of illness and of neuroleptic treatment. These results further support the concept that the blunted response is not due to neuroleptic exposure and are of particular interest because the method for defining negative symptoms used in this study is that used to delineate Type II schizophrenia.

Malas et al. (1987) also found that patients with poor premorbid social function (another longitudinal variable) had a significantly lower GH response than did other schizophrenic patients. Such a group of asocial patients probably overlaps substantially with negative symptom schizophrenia subtypes. Certain issues, however, make interpretation of the Malas et al. study problematic: the unstated rationale for their dichotomization score; the high average GH responses in patients and controls; and the lack of data about the comparability of the two patient groups relative to other features. The relationship between neuroendocrine dysfunction in schizophrenia and the Type I/Type II dichotomy is discussed in greater detail in Chapter 8 by Keshavan et al. in this volume.

Validity of the Deficit Syndrome

In contrast to Type II schizophrenia, the concept of the deficit syndrome assumes psychotic symptoms are orthogonal to primary, enduring negative symptoms, a concept supported by empirical research (Lewine 1985). The deficit-nondeficit dichotomy is exclusively based on the presence or absence of primary, enduring negative symptoms. A study of deficit patients has shown that cross-sectional severity of their psychotic symptoms is similar to that of nondeficit schizophrenic patients (Carpenter et al. 1988).

Deficit patients have also been shown to differ from other chronic schizophrenic patients on a number of measures. The neuropsychological function of clinically stable schizophrenic outpatients (15 with the deficit syndrome and 15 matched nondeficit patients) was compared to that of 15 age- and sex-matched normal control subjects (Wagman et al. 1987). Both schizophrenic groups had significantly lower scores on a psychomotor factor than did control subjects. The deficit syndrome group, but not the nondeficit patients, performed more poorly than normal controls on a general performance factor. The results were not associated with severity of either positive or negative symptoms at the time of testing, but rather depended on the enduring quality of negative symptoms.

In a study by Buchanan et al. (in press), 17 deficit and 17 nondeficit schizophrenic patients matched on the basis of age, race, and gender were administered the Neurological Evaluation Scale, a neurologic signs battery based on a theoretical synthesis of previous work on neurologic impairment in schizophrenia (Buchanan and Heinrichs 1989; Heinrichs and Buchanan 1988). The battery assesses cerebral dominance, frontal release signs, eye movements, synkinetic movements, and three functional areas of interest (i.e., sensory integration, sequencing of complex motor acts, and motor coordination). Deficit patients exhibited more total abnormal findings, as well as a greater impairment of sensory integration.

Although abnormalities of smooth pursuit eye movement (SPEM) have been described in schizophrenic patients, the underlying mechanisms and clinical correlates remain unclear. To explore these issues further, Thaker et al. (1988) carried out eye movement examination in saccade, antisaccade, fixation, and smooth pursuit paradigms in 54 DSM-III schizophrenic outpatients. The order of presentation for these paradigms was randomized. Saccadic distractibility did not correlate with SPEM score, but was significantly associated with tardive dyskinesia ($r = .59$). In contrast, SPEM score and latency for volitional saccades did not correlate with tardive dyskinesia. Latency for volitional saccades significantly differentiated schizophrenic patients with the deficit syndrome from nondeficit patients (356 ± 66 msec versus 299 ± 60, $P < .01$). The short duration of this latency suggests this is not an impairment of voluntary attention. These data also suggest that the abnormality associated with the deficit syndrome does not reflect a generalized performance impairment.

Anhedonia, a lack of the experience of gratification and pleasure, has long been noted to be a key feature of chronic schizophrenia (Kraepelin 1919; Meehl 1962; Rado 1956). Chapman and Chapman (1985) operationalized this concept in two of their "psychosis proneness" scales. These five scales, designed to select those at high risk for the development of psychosis, are physical anhedonia, social anhedonia, impulsive nonconformity, perceptual aberration, and magical ideation. We hypothesized that deficit syndrome patients would, in comparison to nondeficit schizophrenic patients, have higher scores on physical anhedonia and social anhedonia, but would not differ relative to perceptual aberration and magical ideation. Although, anhedonia per se is not a specific item in our definition of the deficit syndrome, it fits conceptually.

Two groups of DSM-III chronic schizophrenic patients were administered the Chapman psychosis proneness scales. The two groups (16 deficit and 42 nondeficit patients) did not differ relative to age, gender distribution, racial composition, or socioeconomic status. As hypothesized, deficit syndrome patients had higher scores on physical anhedonia and social anhedonia, but the two groups did not differ on perceptual aberration, magical ideation, or impulsive nonconformity (Kirkpatrick and Buchanan 1990).

Finally, in an exploratory study with Carol Tamminga (unpublished study), the metabolic activity of cortical and subcortical structures was assessed using positron emission tomography (PET) imaging with [18]fluoro-2-deoxyglucose, revealing significant differences between deficit and nondeficit patients. These preliminary data encourage further PET studies using the deficit-nondeficit dichotomy.

The findings outlined above support the usefulness of the Type I–Type II and deficit-nondeficit schizophrenia distinctions. In choosing between the overlapping Type II and deficit syndrome constructs, investigators may wish to consider the following.

First, Type I–Type II is based on a number of criteria that collectively may enhance the definition of disease entities. One drawback is the emphasis on positive symptoms in the definition of Type I schizophrenia, although the positive symptom process is by definition present in all cases of schizophrenia. The most important drawback, however, is that findings that validate the Type I–Type II distinction may relate to any of the defining criteria, not necessarily to the negative symptom process per se. In the Type I–Type II construct, patients may move from Type I to Type II over time, but Type II is considered irreversible. Comparisons are therefore likely to skew young patients in early phases of illness toward Type I unless specific matching is done. As is so common in the literature, observed differences may relate to age, illness duration, phase of illness, a difference in cross-sectional positive symptom level, or the negative symptom process.

Second, the deficit-nondeficit dichotomy focuses solely on the enduring, primary negative symptom component. It is not a broad definition of a disease entity, but rather a focused approach to one psychopathologic process. Differences between deficit and nondeficit forms of schizophrenia may be related to this process, and matching on potential confounders has already proven feasible.

THE HEURISTIC APPLICATION OF THE DEFICIT CONSTRUCT

Primary negative symptoms represent core psychopathology that is frequently, but not always, observed within the schizophrenia syndrome. As phenomena central to the understanding of schizophrenia, primary negative symptoms can be specifically addressed in their own right. Since this domain of psychopathology is distinguishable from other domains and may have relatively poor within-patient correlations with other domains, there is further reason to believe it is best studied when isolated. It is not necessary to consider the deficit syndrome as occurring only in schizophrenia, as this domain of psychopathology may be present in other diagnostic classes (e.g., schizotypal personality or chronic unremitting forms of affective disorder) and may even provide a basis for reconceptualizing the nosology of psychoses in the future (Carpenter and Stephens 1982). This conceptualization of the importance of deficit features, as opposed to negative symptoms, has several implications.

First, there are virtually no empirical data regarding treatment effects on primary negative symptoms, particularly the trait or enduring form. Failure to isolate this domain in hundreds of clinical trials has left the field uninformed on the specific therapeutic effects of antipsychotic medication (Carpenter 1980; Carpenter et al. 1981). It is clear that negative symptoms in a generic sense improve contemporaneously with improvement in psychosis during antipsychotic drug treatment (Goldberg 1985), but follow-up studies fail to support the contention that the antipsychotic drugs have remarkably altered the long-term course of personality deterioration (Angst 1988; McGlashan 1988). There may be one exception. Bleuler (1968,1978) argued that the acute-onset, devastating course form of illness may occur less frequently today than prior to the introduction of neuroleptic drugs. In contrast to the clinical trial literature, the psychosocial rehabilitation and other long-term clinical care models have attempted to describe changes relevant to primary negative symptoms. The descriptors, however, have been confounded with general functional attributes, such as social participation and occupational functioning, leaving cloudy the issue of whether the primary psychopathology in the deficit domain is altered.

Second, primary negative symptoms provide a far more specific and compelling basis for establishing animal models of the psychopathology of schizophrenia. Wise's (1982) work in establishing the neuroleptic-induced anhedonia model is an interesting case in point.

Third, the study of the etiology of negative symptoms should be distinguished from the study of the etiology of schizophrenia; the several domains of psychopathology may vary in their etiology and pathogenic mechanisms. This contention is clearly articulated in the hypotheses underlying Type I and Type II schizophrenia (Crow 1985). Unless deficit features are specifically addressed, however, the interpretation of studies will be compromised. For example, studies of negative symptoms to date have very often involved comparison of two groups of schizophrenic patients who differed on a number of dimensions other than negative symptoms per se. Such so-called negative symptom patients may be older, more chronic, and later in their course of illness; have fewer positive symptoms; and so on. When differences are found, it is not known whether they relate to the presence of the primary negative symptom psychopathology or to one or more of the other between-group differences.

Fourth, the genetics of the deficit syndrome may be different than the genetics of schizophrenia per se. If this is correct, linkage studies will be dependent on a phenotype defined by primary negative symptoms.

There is now an exciting opportunity to make substantial progress in understanding the etiology, pathogenesis, pathophysiology, and therapeutics of primary negative symptoms. A number of chapters in this volume are devoted to discrete hypotheses relevant to pathophysiology and/or therapeutics. The argument for frontal and prefrontal lobe involvement (and possible underlying mechanisms) has been reviewed in the literature (Carpenter et al. 1985; Levin 1984; Weinberger 1987) and is discussed later in this volume in the section on Structural and Developmental Theories. Several neurotransmitter hypotheses are credible. We have previously reviewed evidence supporting a biogenetic amine depletion hypothesis (Carpenter et al. 1985). Cholinergic, serotonergic, and catecholamine hypotheses are reviewed in this volume in the section on Biochemical Hypotheses.

CONCLUSIONS

Schizophrenia is a heterogeneous clinical syndrome. Defining the core psychopathologic processes is crucial to progress in etiologic and therapeutic research. Kraepelin (1919) initiated this effort, and several domains currently merit attention (Carpenter and Buchanan 1989). Perhaps the most important area of psychopathology is defined by negative symptoms, for these account for the deterioration in personal functioning so devastating in some forms of schizophrenia. It is important, therefore, to have a clear and reliable definition of the negative symptom construct.

Much work to date on negative symptoms is confounded. The main reasons are 1) failure to distinguish primary from secondary symptomatology; 2) failure to distinguish trait from state; 3) conceptualization of positive symptoms as inversely related to negative symptoms; and 4) use of multiple criteria to define contrasting cohorts, making it difficult to identify the source of cohort differences.

We have described an approach explicitly focused on enduring, primary negative symptoms. This approach separates this core pathologic process (the deficit syndrome) for specific study. One can then use this delineation to categorize deficit and nondeficit groups. In comparative studies, patients in these two groups can be similar in other features (e.g., positive symptoms), allowing less confounded study of the negative symptom domain.

APPENDIX

Diagnostic Criteria for the Deficit Syndrome of Schizophrenia

1. At least two of the following six negative symptoms must be present:
   a. restricted affect
   b. diminished emotional range

    c. poverty of speech
    d. curbing of interests
    e. diminished sense of purpose
    f. diminished social drive

2. Some combination of two or more of the negative symptoms listed above have been present for the preceding 12 months and always were present during periods of clinical stability (including chronic psychotic states) or following recovery from psychotic exacerbation. These symptoms may or may not be detectable during transient episodes of acute psychotic disorganization or decompensation.

3. The negative symptoms above are primary (i.e., not secondary to factors other than the disease process). Such factors include:
    a. anxiety
    b. drug effect
    c. suspiciousness (and other psychotic symptoms)
    d. mental retardation
    e. depression

4. The patient meets DSM-III-R criteria for schizophrenia.

Chapter 2

Longitudinal Course of Negative Symptoms in Schizophrenia

Stanley R. Kay, Ph.D.

Chapter 2

Longitudinal Course of Negative Symptoms in Schizophrenia

THE POSITIVE-NEGATIVE DISTINCTION: A MILESTONE IN SCHIZOPHRENIA RESEARCH?

Since the early writings of Bleuler (1950), more than 80 years ago, it has been recognized that schizophrenia is a heterogeneous condition; any attempt to understand it requires explanation of its various guises or components. It is evident to clinicians that patients with schizophrenia differ widely in their symptomatic presentation, premorbid functioning, genetic liability, response to medication, and prognosis.

Such diversity is of more than theoretical interest; it demands that we reconsider the logic behind our principal treatment for schizophrenia: the neuroleptic drug. The use of dopamine-blocking agents for this condition, which originated in the 1950s, best fits a unitary model of schizophrenia, one characterized by dopamine excess in the central nervous system. The limitations of this treatment strategy are revealed, however, by a lack of efficacy for a large segment of patients and in the failure of neuroleptics to reverse many crucial symptoms, even among those who otherwise can be considered responders.

The need for a revised and expanded view of schizophrenia has become increasingly apparent. Based on factorial study, Strauss et al. (1974) proposed that we may recognize two separate symptom profiles in schizophrenia: positive symptoms, consisting of abnormal productions, and negative symptoms, consisting of deficits or loss of

I gratefully acknowledge the vital contributions of colleagues who participated in the research described herein: Lewis A. Opler, M.D., Ph.D.; Abraham Fiszbein, M.D.; Man Mohan Singh, M.D.; Jean-Pierre Lindenmayer, M.D.; Lisa M. Murrill, M.A.; and Victor M. Rosado, M.D.

function. Subsequently, Crow (1980a, 1980b) and Andreasen and colleagues (Andreasen and Olsen 1982; Andreasen et al. 1982) hypothesized that positive symptoms prevail in the acute stage and may represent a hyperdopaminergic state. Patients of this type were thus characterized by a possible neurochemical abnormality that is considered reactive to neuroleptics and portends a good outcome. Negative symptoms, by contrast, were thought to predominate mainly in the chronic stage and perhaps signify structural brain abnormality, such as indicated by ventricular enlargement. Patients of this description were expected to be neuroleptic resistant and to carry a poor prognosis.

This proposition has obvious appeal in its simple dichotomization, rooted in different forms of neuropathology, and in its embrace of much of the diversity seen in schizophrenia. If validated, the model could clarify systematic differences in the etiology, pharmacotherapy, and prognosis of schizophrenia.

Empirical research, unfortunately, has not uniformly supported the principal tenets of the Crow-Andreasen model (Pogue-Geile and Zubin 1988). The experiments by Andreasen and Olsen (1982) and Angrist et al. (1980), often quoted in support of the model, are limited by inadequacies in sampling, and even by results that undermine the interpretations (Opler et al. 1987). For example, Andreasen's negative schizophrenia group was significantly older than the positive one and had far more experience with electroconvulsive treatment (56% versus 5%), which might well account for some of the cognitive and neurologic differences (Friedberg 1961). In the Angrist et al. (1980) study, the conclusion that negative symptoms failed to respond to neuroleptics is tempered by the fact that one of the three negative items assessed (emotional withdrawal) did improve significantly. Subsequent studies on the relationship of negative symptomatology to brain structure, drug response, phase of illness, and prognosis have yielded mixed results that appear to defy this simple categorization (see review by Pogue-Geile and Zubin 1988).

SOURCES OF ERROR VARIANCE: THE BANE OF RESEARCH

This absence of consistent findings, while requiring explanation, may not be reason to discount the validity of the positive-negative distinction. This still young area of research is beset by several fundamental methodological weaknesses, which are likely to augment Type II error (i.e., to militate against consistent findings) (Kay and Opler 1987; Sommers 1985; Zubin 1985). These include inadequacies of rating scales, lack of specificity of the construct investigated, excessive reliance on cross-sectional assessments, limited range of follow-up data, and the absence of drug-free assessments.

To elaborate, the reliance on negative symptom rating scales that are not fully operationalized and standardized may promote measurement that is weak, inaccurate, or simply invalid. For example, the most widely used scales (e.g., Andreasen and Olsen 1982; Heinrichs et al. 1984; Iager et al. 1985; Lewine et al. 1983; Overall and Gorham 1962) provide neither a standardized interview nor specific rating criteria to decide between different levels of symptom severity (e.g., mild versus moderate). These methods also have been criticized for uncertain content and construct validity as well as lack of retest reliability (Kay et al. 1986a; Zubin 1985). Carpenter et al. (1985) persuasively argued that several of the symptoms that have been classified as negative (e.g., attention dysfunction and disorientation) may actually be a consequence of positive features, such as hallucinations or hyperarousal. Investigations at Columbia University (Bilder et al. 1985; Cornblatt et al. 1985) and at our own facility (Kay et al. 1986b, 1986c) also suggest that attentional impairment may cluster equally with negative and positive symptoms. The topic of rating scales is dealt with in greater detail elsewhere (Silk and Tandon, Chapter 4, this volume).

Second, many studies analyze negative symptoms in a vacuum, without due consideration for how they may differ from positive or other symptoms. Unless the phenomena attributed to the negative syndrome are specific and unique to that cluster of symptoms, the conclusions will be grossly misleading, having perhaps more to do with the severity than the character of the disorder. Studies on negative psychopathology, therefore, require a psychometrically comparable measure of other symptoms that serve, in effect, as "controls."

A third methodological concern, of primary interest for this chapter, is the tendency to study negative features cross-sectionally. It is important to recognize that the cross-sectional view is a static one that tells us little about hypothesized processes and, by its very nature, precludes inspection of their stability, course, and mutability over time. Since the negative syndrome has been ascribed specific longitudinal characteristics—prominence in the chronic stage, lack of response to neuroleptics, poor long-term outcome—it is essential that studies of its validity be capable of testing these assumptions.

Fourth, the few investigations that have examined negative symptoms longitudinally have been limited by short-term designs that cover several weeks of neuroleptic treatment, or by retrospective views of the course of illness. For example, the longitudinal studies of Pogue-Geile and Harrow (1984, 1985), although highly informative, were derived from retrospective assessment of negative symptoms rather than from concurrent baseline analysis and subsequent follow-up. We cannot establish the predictive significance of a negative presentation without a prospective design, and we cannot presume truly to know its prognostic import without long-term follow-up.

Finally, the overwhelming majority of studies on the negative syndrome have not investigated patients in a natural, drug-free state. As a result, the observations may be contaminated by prior clinical response to neuroleptics, which will obviously alter the psychiatric picture in specific ways. The very persistence of negative features after drug treatment may, in fact, provide for a self-selected sample in studies that lack a drug-free baseline. Thus one cannot reasonably assume that the negative profile carries the same meaning in a drug-treated as in an unmedicated patient, whose negative symptoms have gone unchallenged and therefore may still subside with the intervention. As has been amply stressed (Carpenter et al. 1985; Rifkin et al. 1975), the assessment of negative symptoms in medicated patients also may be confounded by drug side effects that restrict verbal, motor, and social functions (e.g., akinesia).

To address these methodological pitfalls, our research group has embarked on studies that emphasize use of a well-operationalized syndrome scale, multidimensional assessment, longitudinal study with prospective baseline measures, and either drug-free evaluation or independent ratings for drug side effects. In this chapter, we summarize a series of investigations that separately reflect on the short- and long-term longitudinal course of the negative syndrome. Findings support the reliability and validity of the negative syndrome in schizophrenia as a pathologic process distinct from the positive syndrome and general psychopathology (Kay and Singh 1989; Merriam et al. 1990). The concept of the negative syndrome that emerges, however, does not correspond to the model originally proposed by Crow and Andreasen and seems to differ systematically at different stages of the illness.

ASSESSMENT OF THE NEGATIVE SYNDROME

The validity and scope of one's observations are directly limited by the device used for measurement. This fact is particularly true in studying a new construct, such as the negative syndrome (Zubin 1985). For this reason, we developed and standardized a psychiatric rating scale in accordance with the guidelines for test construction mandated by the American Psychological Association (1974). The result is the 30-item, 7-point Positive and Negative Syndrome Scale (PANSS), which has the following psychometric advantages (Kay et al. 1989): 1) formal criteria for conducting the 30- to 40-minute psychiatric interview, which follows a four-stage sequence for comprehensive assessment; 2) thorough definition of all items at each of seven levels of symptom severity, as contained in the PANSS Rating Manual (Kay et al. 1987b); 3) a standard videotape procedure for training in the PANSS interview and ratings (Kay 1988) to help establish consensus across raters and research groups; 4) content sampling that is balanced, encompasses several functional spheres, and excludes "secondary" negative features; and 5) provision of parallel scales of positive syndrome and general psychopathology to serve as a basis for interpreting the negative syndrome.

The psychometric properties of the PANSS were studied on a total of almost 200 schizophrenic patients to evaluate their reliability, validity, and scaling characteristics (Kay et al. 1987a, 1988). We found the interrater reliabilities between psychiatrist and psychologist on a sample of 31 acute schizophrenic patients to range between .81 and .88 ($P < .0001$). Then, on a sample of 49 chronic schizophrenic patients, we compared our method with that of Andreasen and Olsen (1982) and also against the Clinical Global Impressions Scale (Guy 1976). For all three scales, the corresponding correlations were significant ($P < .0001$), supporting the criterion-related validity of the PANSS (Kay et al. 1988). Finally, we examined the internal consistency, distribution, and interrelationships of the PANSS scales on 101 chronic schizophrenic patients (Kay et al. 1987b). Coefficient alpha was .83 and .73 for the negative and positive scales, respectively, and each of the individual items correlated significantly with the remaining scale total. The three PANSS scales were observed to be normally distributed, without substantial skewness or kurtosis. Although the two syndromes were modestly intercorrelated ($r = .27$, $P < .05$), both were far more strongly related to the general psychopathology scale ($r = .60$ with negative and .68 with positive syndrome, $P < .0001$). The more severely ill patients, therefore, exhibited greater symptoms of both kinds. Once we statistically partialed out the shared variance from severity of illness, however, a significant inverse correlation between the two syndromes emerged ($r = -.23$, $P < .05$). This finding supported the construct validity of the syndromes as essentially non-overlapping, discrete aspects of the schizophrenic disorder.

LONGITUDINAL COURSE IN ACUTE AND CHRONIC SCHIZOPHRENIA

The PANSS was applied to 37 acute schizophrenic patients (22 men) who had been newly admitted to an intake unit of an urban psychiatric center (Lindenmayer et al. 1984). The patients had a mean age of 23.6 years (range, 18–34). For all patients, 2 or fewer years had elapsed since first psychiatric admission (mean, 1.42), and approximately 60% had no or only one prior hospitalization. The baseline data indicated that negative symptoms were as prevalent as positive symptoms and were not secondary to prolonged institutionalization, severity of illness, neuroleptic dose, or drug side effects.

It was possible to follow up 19 patients from this sample for an average period of 2.2 years, reflecting the progression from the acute into the early chronic phase of schizophrenia (Lindenmayer et al. 1986). A comparison of this group with the 18 dropouts suggested equivalence: no differences were found in age, sex, ethnic group, marital status, education, premorbid ratings, age first hospitalized, or baseline severity of illness. When we examined the longitudinal course of the negative and positive syndromes over 2 years, we found no measurable increase or decrease in the means. Similarly, the autocorrelations of the syndromes from baseline to follow-up were nonsignificant, suggesting that the patients were in a state of flux.

The import of the negative and positive syndromes, however, seemed to change radically over this transitional phase. In direct contrast to popular belief, the negative syndrome at index admission predicted not worse but better subsequent functioning (Table 2-1). This finding was indicated by significant correlations with follow-up assessments on seven of the nine items from the Strauss and Carpenter (1972) Multidimensional Outcome Scale, which probes social, occupational, and psychiatric adjustment. Some of the predictive correlations were surprisingly high—for example, the correlation between baseline negative syndrome and follow-up quantity of useful work ($r = .73$, $P < .001$). Whereas a negative syndrome was unrelated to premorbid functioning ($r = -.25$), it was significantly associated with the PANSS depression cluster ($r = .65$, $P < .01$), which too was a predictor of better overall level of functioning at follow-up ($r = .52$, $P < .05$) (Kay and Lindenmayer 1987). A positive syndrome, meanwhile, carried no prognostic significance; however, like the negative syndrome, it reflected greater severity of the concurrent illness when reassessed 2 years later.

Although these data support the predictive validity of a negative syndrome in acute schizophrenia, they of course do not imply that this clinical variable fully or uniquely explains outcome. Premorbid adjustment, a long-established prognosticator for schizophrenia (Phillips 1953), expectedly also showed sizable correlations with overall level of functioning ($r = .47$, $P < .05$) and lower general psychopathology ($r = .54$, $P < .02$) at 2-year follow-up. Because of the nonoverlap between premorbid status and baseline negative

Table 2-1. Predictive and contemporaneous significance of negative and positive syndromes in acute schizophrenia

Outcome criteria	Baseline (predictive r)			Follow-up (contemporaneous r)		
	Negative score	Positive score	Negative-positive difference (P)	Negative score	Positive score	Negative-positive difference (P)
Multidimensional Outcome Scale						
Duration of nonhospitalization	.53*	−.13	<.10	−.20	−.30	
Frequency of social contacts	.39	.04		−.36	−.52*	
Quality of social relations	.48*	.02	<.10	−.45	−.67***	
Quantity of useful work	.73†	.26	<.05	−.56**	−.60***	
Quality of useful work	.61***	−.09	<.01	−.67***	−.68***	
Absence of symptoms	.48*	−.08	<.05	−.61***	−.83†	
Ability to meet own basic needs	.29	.17		−.53*	−.05	
Fullness of life	.59***	.05	<.02	−.71†	−.53*	<.05
Overall level of functioning	.47*	.04	<.10	−.69***	−.69***	
Positive and Negative Syndrome Scale						
General psychopathology	−.30	.01		.70†	.65***	

*P < .05. **P < .02. ***P < .01. †P < .001.
Source. Based on Lindenmayer et al. (1986).

syndrome, however, these predictors combined to produce a significantly stronger multiple correlation with the two outcome measures ($r = .77$, $P < .001$; and $r = .70$, $P < .005$; respectively) (Kay and Lindenmayer 1987).

A parallel longitudinal study was recently completed on a sample of 58 chronic schizophrenic patients drawn from long-term units of the same psychiatric hospital (Kay and Murrill 1990). Of these patients, it was possible to locate 46 (79.3%) for follow-up after a period that averaged 2.7 years. In this investigation, as in the acute study, the follow-up assessments were performed without knowledge of the baseline positive and negative ratings. The present group was predominantly male ($n = 44$), was almost 10 years older than our acute sample (mean age, 33.1 years), and at baseline had a mean of 11.78 years of illness since first hospitalization.

The prognostic analyses provided an interesting contrast to those conducted on patients in the acute stage. As shown in Table 2-2, the PANSS negative syndrome was not significantly associated with better or poorer outcome on the Multidimensional Outcome Scale. The

Table 2-2. Prognostic significance of negative, positive, and general psychopathology symptoms in chronic schizophrenia

Outcome criteria	Positive and Negative Syndrome Scale baseline assessment		
	Negative syndrome	Positive syndrome	General psychopathology
Multidimensional Outcome Scale			
Duration of nonhospitalization	.02	−.37***	−.16
Frequency of social contacts	−.08	−.27	−.21
Quality of social relations	.01	−.16	−.09
Quantity of useful work	−.28	−.30*	−.20
Quality of useful work	−.27	−.14	−.12
Absence of symptoms	−.27	−.28	−.28
Ability to meet own basic needs	−.25	−.10	−.15
Fullness of life	−.09	−.33**	−.18
Overall level of functioning	−.21	−.26	−.21
Days of hospitalization across 1-year interval during follow-up	.04	.35**	.17

*$P < .05$. **$P < .025$. ***$P < .01$.

positive syndrome, however, now carried ominous implications for subsequent functioning on three of the component scales: duration of nonhospitalization, quantity of useful work, and fullness of life. In addition to the rated assessment, the positive syndrome predicted greater number of days of actual inpatient hospitalization during the follow-up term. General psychopathology, like the negative scale, did not significantly predict outcome in the 2.7-year follow-up for this chronic sample.

PHASIC STUDIES OF THE SYNDROMES

Despite the methodological strengths of the longitudinal research design, there are two inherent shortcomings: 1) attrition of subjects, which may affect not only sample size but also its composition, and 2) limited length of follow-up that is feasible. For these reasons, we also pursued a cross-sectional approach for a large-scale phasic study of the negative syndrome (Kay et al. 1986b). The investigation involved 134 schizophrenic inpatients with a mean age of 33.5 years (range, 18–68) who were classified according to the convention of Brown (1960) and others into three stages of the illness: acute (up to 2 years since first hospital admission; mean, .061 years; n = 33), chronic (3–10 years; mean, 6.13; n = 38), and long-term chronic (more than 10 years; mean, 19.78; n = 63). The results are summarized in Table 2-3.

Again, we found no differences in the magnitude of syndrome scores as a function of chronicity, suggesting that there is no evolution toward a greater negative presentation. The PANSS scores were strikingly similar for the acute, chronic, and long-term chronic schizophrenic patients: mean negative scores = 21.4, 21.2, and 23.1, respectively; mean positive scores = 18.8, 19.7, and 18.0, respectively.

Also in keeping with our longitudinal data, the present study found that the import of the syndromes was stage-specific. In acute schizophrenia, a negative score correlated significantly with genealogical and clinical signs of good prognosis—that is, absence of familial psychosis and presence of various atypical and catatonic phenomena, such as expressive immobility, motor retardation, disorientation, and mannerisms and posturing. Quite the reverse profile—one boding poor prognosis—was found for a positive syndrome in the acute stage and, likewise, for a negative syndrome in the chronic stage. These patients had a family history of either less affective disorder or more psychosis. They also had poorer premorbid functioning, as suggested by lesser education and failure to marry. The results on the negative syndrome in chronic schizophrenia were consistent with our earlier typological (Opler et al. 1984) and dimen-

Table 2-3. Covariates of negative and positive syndromes according to chronicity of illness, and tests of significance of the differences

Variables	Partial correlation (r)			Difference between rs (z)		
	Acute	Chronic	Long-term chronic	Acute–chronic	Acute–long-term chronic	Chronic–long-term chronic
Negative syndrome with:						
Familial psychosis	−.30	.09	.40†		3.07***	
Years of education	−.24	−.13	−.29*			
Guilt feelings	−.17	−.44***	−.05			1.98*
Mannerisms & posturing	.25	−.25	.12	1.98*		
Disorientation	.55***	.24	.14		2.10*	
Poor impulse control	.06	.35*	.40†			
Preoccupation	.47***	−.10	.34***	2.37**		
Expressive immobility	.75†	.42***	.51†	2.04*		2.12*
Psychomotor retardation	.47***	.00	.28*	1.97*		

Positive syndrome with:						
Familial affective disorder	-.49***	-.18	-.06		1.99*	
Familial sociopathy	.29	.40**	.06			
Years of education	-.25	.33	.05	2.26*		2.54**
Marital status	.06	.27	-.26*			
Sex (male)	-.33	-.23	.35***		3.07***	2.81***
Guilt feelings	.13	-.29	.20			
Tension	.06	.46***	.48†		2.01*	2.35**
Uncooperativeness	-.20	.48***	.24	2.82***		
Poor attention	.09	.42***	.27*			
Disturbance of volition	.00	.18	.46†		2.15*	
Inappropriate affect	.19	.53†	.42†			
Severity of illness	.39*	.73†	.61†	2.01*		

*P < .05. **P < .02. ***P < .01. †P < .001.
Source. Based on Kay et al. (1986a).

sional studies (Kay et al. 1986c), in which it was associated with lesser education, a more primitive conceptual development, and a family history of "probable schizophrenia" (i.e., schizophrenia or unspecified psychosis that required inpatient treatment). These data on the chronic negative condition also were congruent with findings from independent groups who noted similar relationships between negative symptoms and premorbid deficits (Andreasen and Olsen 1982; Pogue-Geile and Harrow 1984), cognitive impairment (Andreasen and Olsen 1982), and genetic liability (Dworkin and Lenzenweger 1984).

Thus the various research perspectives that we pursued supported the validity of the positive-negative distinction by identifying basic premorbid, developmental, genealogical, and prognostic differences. Our findings were not compatible with the Crow-Andreasen's hypothesis on the negative syndrome, however, because the data challenge the important premises of stability, tendency to worsen over time, and poor prognosis. In fact, if there is a stage specificity, there may be little basis to regard the negative syndrome as a monolithic construct. Only in the chronic negative condition did it appear that a negative presentation may reflect an intransigent, residual deficit picture. In early schizophrenia, a negative syndrome was just as prominent but carried the opposite implications for prognosis. Indeed, it also was associated with a more favorable genealogical profile and with two phenomenological predictors of good outcome: depressive features and atypical catatonic symptoms. Either manifestation can produce a negative-like state consisting of diminished affect, slowed motorium, and social isolation.

NEGATIVE SYNDROME IN THE DRUG-FREE STATE

One could hypothesize from the foregoing data that the "true" negative syndrome is a phenomenon that arises only in the chronic phase. Indeed, the negative profile in acute schizophrenia may conceivably represent a "pseudonegative" syndrome comprised of depressive and/or catatonic symptoms. Alternative possibilities are that the chronic negative picture is simply the visible residue in treatment nonresponders, or that we are witnessing an iatrogenic end state rather than a genuine deficit. To tease apart these explanations clearly requires a prospective, drug-free design with long-term longitudinal follow-up. Only with such methodological controls can one be confident that the data reflect on the natural state and course of the illness, uncontaminated by neuroleptic effects.

With this aim, we pooled data from four earlier inpatient psychopharmacologic studies that had been conducted on a closed research unit of a large state psychiatric hospital (Singh and Kay 1975a, 1975b, 1976; Singh and Smith 1973). The combined sample included 62 schizophrenic patients (38 women) who had been screened according to the narrow British diagnostic system of Slater and Roth (1969); the data collection antedated the Research Diagnostic Criteria (Spitzer et al. 1978) and DSM-III (American Psychiatric Association 1980). The sample was generally young, in the subacute phase, and fairly well balanced in gender, ethnic composition, and diagnostic subtype. Patients had a mean age of 25.2 years (range, 18–47) and a mean of 2.9 years since first hospital admission, with only six patients having been ill for more than 5 years. Combined analysis was possible because all four studies used comparable assessments, similar populations, and a within-subjects research design, whereby patients served as their own controls.

The studies consisted of a 1- to 2-week drug washout, followed by 2 to 3 weeks on a drug-free placebo baseline. Patients then received, in double-blind fashion, an individually titrated therapeutic dose of either chlorpromazine or haloperidol, averaging 15 mg daily in haloperidol equivalence. This drug phase lasted 14 to 18 weeks, depending on the particular protocol. Patients were then transferred to another unit or, if sufficiently improved, discharged to the community. Of the 62 patients, 54 (87%) were followed up for 3 years to determine at what point, if at all, they had to be rehospitalized.

Symptoms were assessed prospectively in the placebo baseline and again after the neuroleptic phase, using the Brief Psychiatric Rating Scale (Overall and Gorham 1962) and Psychopathology Rating Schedule (Singh and Kay 1975a). Since these scales were the precursors of the PANSS, we were able to calculate positive and negative syndrome scores post hoc, applying the same item combinations as for the PANSS. The sum of 32 individual symptoms provided a measure of total psychopathology.

Four outcome criteria were applied. First, neuroleptic response was gauged as the degree of improvement in total psychopathology from baseline to final neuroleptic week. Second, residual disorder was the total psychopathology score at the final neuroleptic week. Third, functional reconstitution was judged after the neuroleptic phase by the 5-point Therapy Outcome Rating Scale (Singh and Kay 1979a), which measures final disposition in terms of how fully the patient is restored to premorbid levels of social and emotional adjustment. Fourth, sustained recovery was quantified as the number of months after treatment until hospital readmission, with a range from 0 (never discharged) to 36 (still in the community after 36 months).

STABILITY, INDEPENDENCE, AND PROGNOSTIC IMPORT

These prospective drug-free data were applied to assess the longitudinal stability, independence, and prognostic significance of negative and positive syndromes in schizophrenia (Kay and Singh 1989). First we examined short-term stability during the 2-week drug-free baseline (Table 2-4). High correlations from the end of placebo weeks 1 to 2 were found for both the negative ($r = .78$, $P < .001$) and positive syndrome ($r = .83$, $P < .001$). Paired t tests revealed no significant changes during this brief time.

To examine longer-range stability, we compared the initial drug-free week with the final neuroleptic week, 3 to 4 months later. As indicated in Table 2-4, the correlations for negative and positive syndromes were .43 and .37, respectively (i.e., still significant despite the longer interval and the neuroleptic intervention). The 35% improvement in negative syndrome with neuroleptic treatment was highly significant ($P < .001$) but not as impressive as the gains in positive syndrome (52%) or total psychopathology (46%). The difference between reduction in negative versus positive scores was marginally significant ($P = .06$).

Table 2-4. Stability and changes in syndromal and total psychopathology scales during drug-free baseline and after 14 to 18 weeks on neuroleptics

Basis for comparison	Spectrum of psychopathology		
	Negative	Positive	Total (item mean)
Drug-free baseline ($n = 27$)			
Week 1 mean ± SD	20.9 ± 10.85	17.7 ± 6.01	2.05 ± .61
Week 2 mean ± SD	21.3 ± 9.35	16.7 ± 6.68	2.06 ± .52
Change: mean/%	.4/+ 1.9	− 1.0/− 5.6	.01/+ .5
Significance: paired t	.34	.70	.32
Correlation: Pearson t	.78***	.83***	.72***
Drug-free versus final neuroleptic week ($n = 62$)			
Week 1 mean ± SD	22.6 ± 8.97	20.0 ± 6.66	2.36 ± .74
Final week mean ± SD	14.7 ± 7.82	9.7 ± 7.22	1.28 ± .78
Change: mean/%	− 7.9/− 35.0	− 10.3/− 51.5	− 1.08/− 45.8
Significance: paired t	6.85***	10.34***	9.34***
Correlation: Pearson t	.43***	.37**	.27*

*$P < .05$. **$P < .005$. ***$P < .001$.
Source. Based on Kay and Singh (1989).

To assess the independence or relatedness of the syndromes, we performed intercorrelations during both the drug-free and final neuroleptic week. The finding of note was that negative and positive scores were initially unrelated ($r = .06$), but they were strongly intercorrelated after neuroleptic stabilization ($r = .52$, $P < .001$). Other analyses during the drug-free state again revealed that chronicity of illness (years since first hospital admission) was not associated with negative ($r = .13$) or positive syndrome ($r = .08$).

Finally, we analyzed the drug-free baseline data in relation to four separate outcome criteria to study short-term and longer-range prognosis (Table 2-5). We found that higher drug-free negative and positive syndromes both predicted greater reduction in total psychopathology after 3 to 4 months of neuroleptic treatment. This could possibly represent a "regression to the mean," whereby patients with severer baseline illness have the greater opportunity for improvement. In fact, high scores on both syndromes also were associated with a greater degree of remaining symptoms after treatment, which implies that they convey a poor prognosis.

Where the two syndromes differed was in regard to functional reconstitution and sustained recovery. These results were consistent with our other follow-up studies but ran counter to the common expectation on the positive-negative distinction. We found that the drug-free positive syndrome predicted significantly poorer outcome as judged by more substantial and longer-range criteria. It alone correlated with less complete functional reconstitution after neurolep-

Table 2-5.   Prognostic significance (Pearson r) of negative and positive syndromes in drug-free schizophrenic patients

| | | | Drug-free baseline measure | | |
Outcome criteria	Observation period (months)	n	Negative syndrome	Positive syndrome	Total psychopathology
Neuroleptic response	3–4	62	.28*	.25*	.55†
Residual disorder	3–4	62	.26*	.28*	.27*
Functional reconstitution	3–4	62	−.14	−.32**	−.28*
Months to relapse	36	54	−.08	−.37***	−.35***

*$P < .05$. **$P < .02$. ***$P < .01$. †$P < .005$.
Source.   Based on Kay and Singh (1989).

tic treatment and also with an earlier relapse across the 3-year follow-up. Severity of total psychopathology yielded a similar prognostic pattern as the positive syndrome.

CONCLUSIONS

Our work to date may be summarized as follows.

The negative and positive syndromes are highly stable for the short term in the drug-free state.

They appear to be reasonably stable even after 3 to 4 months of neuroleptic intervention, and despite marked clinical improvements. Stability across a far longer interval, such as 2 years, seems to be uncertain, particularly early in the course of schizophrenia.

In response to neuroleptics, both syndromes are significantly improved from baseline, even though the reduction in negative symptoms is marginally less. These observations are consistent with other recent reports on neuroleptic effect on negative and positive dimensions of schizophrenia (Breier et al. 1987; Johnstone et al. 1987; Meltzer et al. 1986; Tandon et al. 1990b), which conclude that neither group of symptoms is entirely irreversible. Although such findings are compatible with the premise that a positive syndrome represents neurochemical abnormality (i.e., dopamine excess), they challenge the more pessimistic view that the negative syndrome reflects structural deficit and thus is unamenable to neuroleptic treatment.

As to the question of whether the two syndromes are mutually independent, the literature has been quite contradictory. Findings cover the full range from significant direct intercorrelation (Kay et al. 1986c) to no correlation (Johnstone et al. 1987; Lewine et al. 1983) to inverse correlation (Andreasen and Olsen 1982). We previously have argued (Kay and Opler 1987) that the diversity in reports could stem from lack of control for general psychopathology, which covaries with both syndromes (Breier et al. 1987; Kay et al. 1987a) and could mediate their intercorrelation. As these drug-free data show, however, control for neuroleptic status is essential as well. We found a significant correlation between syndromes when patients were stabilized on neuroleptics but no correlation in the natural, drug-free state. This would suggest that the negative and positive syndromes are theoretically independent (i.e., separate constructs), even though in practice they often occur together. It would also suggest that a purer assessment of these independent constructs may be obtained from the drug-free state, notwithstanding the significant predrug to postdrug correlations.

In both our cross-sectional and longitudinal studies, we found no association between chronicity of illness and syndrome scores. Comparably high negative and positive ratings were observed at all phases of the illness: acute, chronic, and long-term chronic. The results challenge the view that positive symptoms prevail in early schizophrenia whereas negative symptoms increasingly dominate as the illness advances.

The two syndromes differ on a broad range of external covariates that may reflect on pathogenesis, such as premorbid status, family history of psychiatric illness, and cognitive profile. The direction of these differences in acute schizophrenia, however, runs counter to the prevailing notion, indicating a more benign rather than less benign process for patients with a pronounced negative picture.

Most strikingly, our prognostic analyses also challenge the assumption that a negative syndrome bodes poor outcome. In early schizophrenia, a negative presentation actually presaged a favorable course. Our prospective drug-free analyses on mostly subacute schizophrenic patients as well as our follow-up of a chronic population found that a worse long-range outcome was anticipated by a higher baseline positive syndrome. For the short term, however, more severe psychopathology of either description predicted greater symptom reduction with neuroleptics but also greater remaining illness. Accordingly, these data suggested that the prognostic import of the syndromes may vary with both phase of illness and time of follow-up assessment.

We conclude, then, that the negative and positive dimensions in schizophrenia may indeed reflect stable, distinct, and fundamental processes that transcend the artifacts of drug side effects and can be reliably measured. Their import seems somewhat at odds with the seminal models of Crow (1980a) and Andreasen and Olsen (1982) and defies a simple unitary model. Nevertheless, there is reason to believe that the positive-negative distinction can explain some of the heterogeneity of schizophrenia. This is not to say, of course, that it can accommodate the full diversity of schizophrenia, nor that it provides the same information as from biological and course-related measures and as from other phenomenological variables. Rather, as we have proposed (Singh and Kay 1987), a better understanding of this disorder may require considering how the positive-negative distinction interacts with other crucial typologies in schizophrenia, such as the acute–chronic (supra), the good versus poor premorbid type (Kay and Lindenmayer 1987), the process–reactive, and the paranoid–nonparanoid.

Clearly, research is still in its infancy and progress depends on clarifying important directions for further exploration. At this point, negative and positive symptom assessment seems to offer the practicing clinician a means of identifying systematic and fundamental distinctions within this multifarious condition. The ultimate hope is that a better understanding of the complex presentation will lead to more rational, individually tailored treatments for schizophrenia.

Chapter 3

Negative Symptomatology in Schizophrenia: Syndrome and Subtype Status

Michael F. Pogue-Geile, Ph.D.
Matcheri Keshavan, M.D.

Chapter 3

Negative Symptomatology in Schizophrenia: Syndrome and Subtype Status

The role that negative symptoms, such as poverty of speech and flat affect, may play in schizophrenia has received considerable research attention in recent years (for reviews see, Kay and Opler 1987; Pogue-Geile and Zubin 1988; Walker and Lewine 1988). Throughout much of this work, the terms *syndrome* and *subtype* are used frequently, and sometimes confusingly. For example, Crow (1980a) initially hypothesized that negative symptoms in schizophrenia represented a behavioral syndrome that was the manifestation of unspecified structural brain abnormalities. In his initial writings, Crow did not directly address the issue of the etiologic subtype status of negative symptoms. In contrast, Andreasen and Olsen (1982) proposed "subtyping" schizophrenia according to the joint occurrence of positive symptoms (e.g., hallucinations and delusions) and negative symptoms into pure positive, pure negative, mixed, and neither symptom subgroups. Since the concepts of syndrome and subtype are central in research on negative symptoms, we seek here to clarify some of the definitional and conceptual issues involved and to review briefly the empirical evidence relevant to them. Definitional and conceptual issues will be considered first.

SYNDROMES AND SUBTYPES: DEFINITIONS AND CONCEPTS

Syndromes

As commonly used, the term *syndrome* differs primarily from *subtype* in its level of analysis. A putative syndrome refers to differences among

Completion of this manuscript was supported in part by grants NIH-BRSG-RR07084 and NIMH-MH43666 to the first author.

symptoms and signs, whereas a hypothesized subtype refers to etiologic differences among individuals within a broader group. Although usually originating from clinical observation, a syndrome may be formally defined as two or more observed characteristics that tend to co-occur more (or less) often than would be expected by chance alone. Before turning to a description of the subtype concept, some aspects of the syndrome concept will be addressed in detail.

First, the constituent characteristics of a putative syndrome may themselves be either dichotomously or quantitatively scaled. For example, the characteristics of poverty of speech and flatness of affect are often scaled quantitatively in terms of their severity, although for some purposes they may be dichotomized into present and absent. Similarly, a syndrome may itself be categorical or quantitative. Although syndromes are usually thought of as being either present or absent, they may also be present in varying degrees. In this case, there is little difference between a quantitatively scaled syndrome and a psychometric dimension, such as that derived from factor analysis. For example, a negative symptom syndrome might be considered as present based on a cutoff score from an additive scale, or alternatively, individuals might be ranked according to their additive scale score into those showing more or less negative symptomatology. Although it may be preferable to use the term *negative symptom dimension* in the latter case, it should be clear that the practical difference between a syndrome and a dimension is generally slight. Furthermore, a syndrome either may or may not be hypothesized to be stable over time in an individual. Most syndromes in general medicine vary over time.

The relationship and overlap between different presumed syndromes is of particular importance for the current discussion. Thus two hypothesized syndromes, such as schizophrenia and the negative symptom syndrome, may be associated positively, negatively, or not at all. A positive association would suggest that the two syndromes tend to co-occur at greater than chance levels. In this case, the strongest positive association would be one in which negative symptoms occur among all and only schizophrenic patients, whereas a weaker positive association would indicate that negative symptoms are more common among schizophrenic than nonschizophrenic subjects, but that not all schizophrenic patients experience them whereas some nonschizophrenic subjects do. A significant association between two syndromes may suggest some common causal factors and is relevant to the concept of a subtype discussed below.

Subtypes

The term *subtype* differs from *syndrome* in several ways. First, a subtype implies a hierarchical relationship between two classificatory schema.

That is, subtypes are nested within some broader category, such as a hypothesized negative symptom subtype of schizophrenia. Second, a subtype refers to individual differences within this broader group. To be considered a subtype, for example, only some, not all, schizophrenic patients should show negative symptoms. Third, a subtype generally has hypothesized etiologic implications for the broader phenomenon. A subtype therefore may be defined as an observed individual difference within some broader group that is hypothesized to delineate a subgroup of individuals who differ from the others in their etiology of the broader phenomenon. This notion of a subtype has stronger theoretical implications than does that of a syndrome. Although the term *subtype* is also sometimes used in an informal fashion to describe differences among individuals within a broader group that do not imply hypothetical etiologic differences, the former definition will be used throughout this discussion.

Either a single or a combination of several observable characteristics may serve as an indicator of a hypothesized etiologic subtype. For instance, the presence of a syndrome may itself serve to define a hypothesized subtype. As was the case for a syndrome, the individual observed indicators, as well as the hypothesized subtype itself, may be either dichotomous or quantitative in nature. Again, although a subtype implies by its name a categorical quality, it may theoretically also be present in varying degrees, as is the case for essential hypertension. Likewise, it could be hypothesized that the degree of negative symptomatology reflects quantitative etiologic differences among schizophrenic patients. Furthermore, although a subtype describes a subgroup of individuals with a hypothesized stable distinct etiology, the observed indicator itself need not necessarily be stable over time.

A subtype, therefore, is a special kind of an individual difference within a broader group. What makes it special is not that a subtype has an etiology of its own (as must any individual difference), but that the etiology of the subtype also determines at least some of the defining characteristics of the broader category. For example, one would not generally consider schizophrenia with negative symptoms as an etiologic subtype of schizophrenia if the etiology of negative symptoms could not also produce the psychotic symptoms that are required for the diagnosis of schizophrenia in those patients who also have negative symptoms. If this were not the case, then negative symptoms might be considered a clinically important difference among patients, but it would no more mark an etiologic subtype of schizophrenia than would differences among patients in height. Therefore, to place our empirical review of the subtype status of negative symptoms in a broader context, we will first consider models of how individual differences in general might arise within a broader group. Of the four such general models that are described below (e.g., Pogue-Geile and Zubin 1988), only some fit the traditional notion of an etiologic subtype.

MODELS OF SUBGROUPING

Independent Influence Model

One alternative, the independent influence model, hypothesizes a trait that may co-occur by chance with a more specific liability to schizophrenia, although the independent trait does not itself contribute to the risk for schizophrenia. For example, a trait, such as asociality, may not contribute to the risk for schizophrenia, but may provide a negative symptom coloring to the presentation when it occurs among schizophrenic patients. It must be recalled that behavioral patterns vary widely in the general population, and that some extremes may be quite similar to negative symptoms typically observed among schizophrenic patients. This model would predict statistical independence between negative symptoms and schizophrenia, which implies that negative symptoms would be equally common among all diagnostic categories and in the general population. In this hypothetical model, negative symptom schizophrenia would not represent an etiologic subtype because, although negative symptoms have their own etiology, it is unrelated to that for other symptoms of schizophrenia.

A special case of this independent influence model that has particular relevance for negative symptoms, positive psychotic symptoms, and diagnostic categories is illustrated in Figure 3-1. In this model, a hypothetical negative symptom liability dimension is theorized to be statistically independent of a presumed positive symptom liability dimension. Thus some psychotic patients will show negative symptoms, some will not, and likewise for individuals with positive symptoms. Furthermore, these dimensions are hypothesized to map onto current diagnostic categories. Using current criteria, individuals 1) high on both dimensions would be diagnosed as schizophrenic; 2) low on both dimensions diagnosed as not ill; 3) high on the negative dimension and low on the positive dimension diagnosed as schizoid; and 4) low on the negative but high on the positive dimension diagnosed as having good prognosis schizophrenia, schizophreniform disorder, atypical psychosis, brief reactive psychosis, or cycloid psychosis. Individuals who are moderate on both the negative symptom dimension and the positive symptom dimension would be diagnosed as schizotypal, which is characterized by both asociality and mild psychotic-like experiences. Although the two negative and positive dimensions are hypothesized to be statistically independent, the negative symptom dimension would become positively associated with the diagnosis of schizophrenia due to current diagnostic practices, according to which some signs of chronicity, in addition to psychotic symptoms, are required to establish the diagnosis (see Correlated Specific Influence Model, Figure 3-1).

If both negative and positive symptom liability dimensions are hypothesized to be largely genetically determined, several predictions follow from this model. First, it would predict, as has been found (e.g., Baron et al. 1985; Kety 1987), an excess of negative symptomatology (i.e., schizoid and schizotypal personality disorders) in the relatives of chronic schizophrenic probands, but not in the relatives of "good prognosis" schizophrenic patients. Similarly, one would expect an excess of psychosis in relatives of chronic schizophrenic probands, but not among relatives of schizoid and schizotypal probands, as was found by Torgerson (1985). Thus relatives of chronic schizophrenic probands would be predicted to be

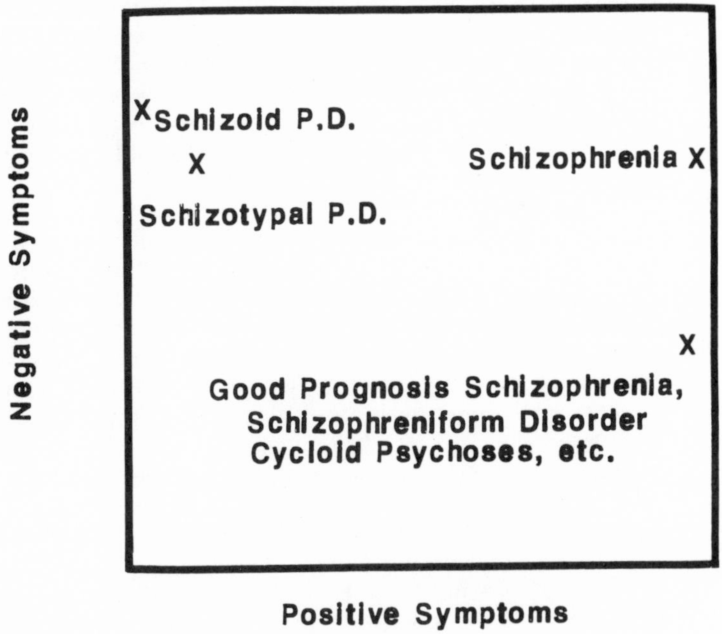

Figure 3-1. Positive and negative symptoms, schizophrenia, and related disorders: The independent influence model.

at increased risk for schizoid-schizotypal disorders, good prognosis schizophrenia, and least commonly for their combination, chronic schizophrenia. In contrast, relatives of schizoid-schizotypal probands would be hypothesized to be at elevated risk for only schizoid-schizotypal disorders, and similarly, relatives of good prognosis schizophrenia would be at risk only for good prognosis schizophrenia, as has been reported by Kety et al. (1978).

Independent Interacting Influence Model

A second general hypothetical model, the independent interacting influence model, proposes that an independent trait, which itself does not contribute to the risk of schizophrenia, interacts with a more specific schizophrenic diathesis. In this model, an independent trait, such as low intelligence, does not contribute to the risk for schizophrenia, but when it occurs among schizophrenic patients, it becomes exacerbated and transformed into a negative symptom picture. Thus only a subset of those schizophrenic patients who are at the extremes of such relevant independent dimensions would develop negative symptoms. In contrast, persons at the extremes of these dimensions who develop nonschizophrenic disorders (e.g., anxiety) would not develop negative symptoms, because an interaction with a schizophrenic liability would be required for the evolution of severe negative symptoms. In this hypothetical model too, negative symptoms would not mark an etiologic subtype of schizophrenia.

Multifactorial Multiple-Threshold Model

A third alternative is the multifactorial, multiple-threshold model (e.g., Reich et al. 1972), in which no etiologic agent (either genetic or environmental) would be a specific cause of negative symptoms. Rather, only the number of etiologic agents contributing to the liability to schizophrenia would determine the occurrence of negative symptomatology, not any specific agent. This multiple-threshold concept can be illustrated in the context of the following hypothesized multifactorial model of schizophrenia. Suppose that five etiologic agents (either genes or experiences) can contribute to the liability to schizophrenia (e.g., agents A, B, C, D, and E), that any three are sufficient to produce diagnosable schizophrenia, and that any four are required to produce schizophrenia with negative symptoms. Alternatively, negative symptom schizophrenia could also be hypothesized to represent an etiologically less severe form of schizophrenia. In this multiple-threshold model, negative symptom schizophrenia does represent an etiologic subtype of schizophrenia, but in a quantitative sense, not in the usual qualitative sense.

Correlated Specific Influence Model

The correlated specific influence model implies that some negative symptom-specific influence is sufficient to produce both negative symptoms and also the generally accompanying positive psychotic symptoms of schizophrenia. Continuing with the hypothetical multifactorial model used above, such an alternative can be illustrated as follows. Suppose again that five etiologic agents (either genetic or environmental) can contribute to the liability to schizophrenia (e.g., A, B, C, D, and E), that any three are sufficient to produce diagnosable schizophrenia, and that agent A also produces negative symptoms. Thus any person with a set of three factors that includes agent A would present with negative symptoms, whereas those without A would not. In the extreme case in which gene or experience A, the negative symptom-specific influence, were sufficient alone to produce both negative symptoms and the psychotic symptoms that are required for the diagnosis of schizophrenia, then negative symptoms would delineate a subtype of schizophrenia with an etiology entirely distinct from that of other schizophrenic patients. This special circumstance is usually what is meant by an etiologic subtype. Even in the multifactorial case, negative symptoms could be said to mark a subtype of schizophrenia whose etiology would differ in some fashion from other patients, although many etiologic factors would also be shared between subtypes.

Summary

These four models of the etiology of individual differences within a broader group provide a general conceptual context for what is meant by the term *subtype* and point the way to strategies for empirically distinguishing among the different possibilities (see Pogue-Geile and Harrow 1987a for further discussion of the empirical predictions from these models). After an examination of the syndrome status of negative symptoms, we will turn to a consideration of the evidence for their status as a subtype.

NEGATIVE SYMPTOMATOLOGY: A SYNDROME?

Methodological Constraints and Empirical Evidence

Evaluation of the syndrome status of negative symptomatology raises a number of methodological concerns. Of primary importance is the definition of negative symptomatology itself. Operational definitions determining which characteristics are included as negative symptoms vary widely (Pogue-Geile and Zubin 1988). As one example, whereas Crow (1985) included only poverty of speech, flat affect, and psychomotor retardation in his definition, Iager et al. (1985) also included memory, orientation, and grooming deficits. It is therefore extremely difficult to evaluate the syndrome status of "negative symptomatology" in general, when such definitional variation prevails across studies. This issue is reviewed in a subsequent chapter on rating scales.

A second important factor is the composition of the study sample. Since the definition of a syndrome involves covariation among characteristics, the amount of variation observed in the constituent characteristics (e.g., flat affect) is important and is undoubtedly influenced by the nature of the subject sample. Findings of covariation are thus sample dependent. To date, almost all of the studies of negative symptomatology have employed only schizophrenic patients as their subjects. These studies therefore depend on and reflect individual differences among schizophrenic patients in negative symptomatology. Rather than assessing the syndrome status of negative symptomatology in some general sense, such studies actually evaluate the status of a negative symptom "subsyndrome," which is nested within the broader syndrome of schizophrenia. Furthermore, the age, sex, chronicity (time since onset of clinical symptoms), and phase of disorder (acute episode or stabilized) characteristics of these schizophrenic samples undoubtedly have some effect on the degree of covariation among negative symptoms. For example, the vast majority of studies to date have assessed inpatients during an acute episode.

Studies of covariation among characteristics also depend on a number of other psychometric factors. First, since detection of the covariation among characteristics is limited by their individual measurement reliabilities, reliability coefficients must be demonstrated to be high for any specific study. Most studies conform to this requirement. Furthermore, ratings of the individual negative symptoms should be blind to eliminate potential rater bias. Without this precaution, apparent covariation among negative symptoms may primarily represent the theoretical preconceptions of the raters. No studies to date have incorporated this methodological precaution. Similarly, shared method variance may also inappropriately inflate observed covariation among negative symptoms. Most assessments of negative symptoms depend on several ratings of observed behavior, which by the nature of the measurement process alone may all tend to covary, regardless of their specific content. In their classic paper on this topic, Campbell and Fiske (1959) advocated a multimethod, multi-trait approach in which the same trait is measured by different methods and different traits are measured by the same methods. To date, no

study has explicitly employed this strategy in investigating the covariation of negative symptomatology.

With these methodological considerations in mind, we will briefly
review studies that have reported either item intercorrelations or
measures of internal consistency for negative symptom scales. Information from the eight studies that have provided such data for current
negative symptom scales is presented in Table 3-1. As can be seen,
although there is some variation across studies, they are unanimous
in showing that negative symptoms tend to correlate positively and
significantly with one another, suggesting the cross-sectional existence among schizophrenic patients of a negative symptom syndrome,
even when defined in a variety of fashions. In addition to the core
symptoms of poverty of speech, flat affect, and psychomotor retardation, some of these scales also include other deficits ranging from
attention and memory to social functioning. At this time, the data are

Table 3-1. Internal consistency of negative symptom scales
among schizophrenic patients

Reference	Scale	Sample N	Cronbach alpha	Average intercorrelation	
				Mean	Range
Andreasen (1982)	SANS	26	.89		
Andreasen and Olsen (1982)	SANS	52		.55	.15–.84
Bilder et al. (1985)	SANS	30		.54	.36–.79
Kulhara et al. (1986)	SANS	98		.55	.44–.70
Moscarelli et al. (1987)	SANS	59		.37	.05–.60
Thiemann et al. (1987)	SANS	35	.80	.50	.26–.64
Pogue-Geile and Harrow (1984)	NSBRS	39	.81	.52	.36–.60
Iager et al. (1985)	NSRS	33		.58	.53–.64
Kay et al. (1987)	PANSS	101	.83		

Note. SANS = Scale for the Assessment of Negative Symptoms. NSBRS = Negative
Symptom Behavior Rating Scale. NSRS = Negative Symptom Rating Scale.
PANSS = Positive and Negative Syndrome Scale.

mixed on whether or not these additional deficits may intercorrelate less strongly with the core negative symptoms. More work needs to be done on defining the further boundaries of the negative symptom construct.

Overall then, these data strongly suggest that a negative symptom syndrome composed of at least flat affect, poverty of speech, and perhaps psychomotor retardation does exist among some schizophrenic patients. There is also evidence for the existence of a broader syndrome, although its further boundaries are not yet clear. In addition, although few studies have attempted to analyze statistically the distribution of negative symptom scores in patient populations, it is usually unimodal and not bimodal. This observation suggests that the negative syndrome might be best thought of as a quantitative dimension, rather than a dichotomous category. Finally, all these studies indicate that a negative symptom syndrome characterizes only a subset of schizophrenic patients at any single cross-sectional assessment. Although generally well supported, these conclusions rest on studies that have a range of weaknesses (as summarized above).

The Negative Symptom Syndrome: A Role Also for Positive Symptoms in Classification?

Although most studies in the area classify schizophrenic patients in a univariate fashion according to the degree of their negative symptomatology alone, some employ a bivariate approach based on the joint cross-sectional profile of negative and positive symptoms, such as delusions and hallucinations (e.g., Andreasen 1982, 1985). This strategy classifies schizophrenic patients based on a cross-sectional assessment into four mutually exclusive categories: positive symptoms predominant, negative symptoms predominant, both symptoms significant, and neither symptom important. It should be noted that this cross-sectional classification scheme differs from the two-dimensional model depicted in Figure 3-1, which refers to the experience of negative and positive symptoms at any point in an individual's lifetime.

The essence of this bivariate approach is that it predicts not only main effects for positive and negative symptoms on various validating characteristics, but also significant interaction effects. Despite this, studies taking this bivariate approach rarely investigate interactions statistically.

Of the many studies that categorize schizophrenic patients into negative or positive groups, only nine reports have exhaustively classified schizophrenic patients based on their joint positive-negative profile (Andreasen and Olsen 1982; Green and Walker 1985, 1986a, 1986b; Kulhara et al. 1986; Moscarelli et al. 1987; Pogue-Geile and Harrow 1984, 1985, 1987a). Most studies omit patients from analyses who have both symptoms or neither. Of these nine reports, all but three (Pogue-Geile and Harrow 1984, 1985, 1987a) included as "mixed" both those patients who have either both or neither symptom, thus making the analysis of interaction effects impossible. Based on these reports that categorically classified patients on their joint positive-negative profile, only two tested statistically the interaction hypothesis, and both found no significant effects (Pogue-Geile and Harrow 1985, 1987a). Of the seven reports that did not explicitly test for interactions, only Andreasen and Olsen reported a large number of significant differences between mixed and negative symptom patients with regard to clinical, biological, and sociodemographic characteristics.

Three reports have taken the dimensional approach of calculating a difference score between negative and positive scores as an attempt to investigate this interactional issue (Andreasen et al. 1982; Kay et al. 1986b, 1986c). This approach has the disadvantage that such difference scores tend to be highly correlated with the individual scores, thus confusing interaction and main effects. With this caveat in mind, a positive-negative difference score was found to be significantly associated with ventricular brain ratio by Andreasen et al. (1982)—same sample as Andreasen and Olsen (1982)—and a variety of symptom and cognitive measures by Kay et al. (1986b, 1986c). The most appropriate dimensional approach to this question has been taken by Green and Walker (1985, 1986a, 1986b), who computed an interaction term and used it in multiple regression analyses. This positive-negative interaction term was not significantly associated with backward masking measures, neuropsychological tests, and attentional tasks. Thus the empirical data thus far have not been particularly supportive of the cross-sectional bivariate approach.

Furthermore, this strategy also generally assigns great importance to the cross-sectional appearance of patients. Since all patients who are diagnosed as schizophrenic must have experienced positive psychotic symptoms at some time to meet current diagnostic criteria, schizophrenic patients with negative symptoms only have by definition experienced positive symptoms in the past. Thus the distinction between negative symptom only and mixed symptom patients may primarily depend on when the assessments were performed.

Finally, this joint positive-negative classification strategy appears to imply that negative and positive symptoms should be negatively correlated with each other—that is, the presence of negative symptoms should decrease the probability of positive symptoms occurring and vice versa. If this were not so, then why should both symptoms be used in classification? Of the 15 studies of the cross-sectional relationship between positive and negative symptoms, only 1 has found them to be significantly negatively correlated (Andreasen and Olsen 1982). In contrast, 12 have found nonsignificant correlations (suggesting statistical independence) (Bilder et al. 1985; Green and Walker 1985; Johnstone et al. 1981; Kulhara and Chadda 1987; Lenzenweger et al. 1989; Lewine et al. 1983; Liddle 1987a; Linden-mayer et al. 1986; Losonczy et al. 1986a, 1986b; Pogue-Geile and Harrow 1984, 1987a; Rosen et al. 1984), and 2 have reported significant positive correlations (Kay et al. 1986b, 1988). Overall, these findings suggest that positive and negative symptoms are generally statistically independent in cross-section, so that all combinations of the two would occur at chance levels. Such statistical independence of the cross-sectional syndromes provides discriminant validity, suggesting that the two should be differentiated and that each can be considered independently of the other. These data thus also imply that classifying patients based on the joint positive-negative symptom profile may not be useful.

In summary, what evidence is available generally weighs against the classification of patients based on the joint profile of positive and negative symptoms. Although more study is needed to be entirely confident of this interpretation, in the absence of a strong theoretical or empirical basis, the added complexity of this bivariate classification scheme does not seem to be more useful than classification based on the degree of negative symptomatology alone.

THE NEGATIVE SYMPTOM SYNDROME: AN ETIOLOGIC SUBTYPE OF SCHIZOPHRENIA?

The evidence reviewed above suggests that at least the core negative symptoms do tend to form a coherent cross-sectional syndrome among some schizophrenic patients. It also seems clear that only a subset of currently diagnosed schizophrenic patients experience marked negative symptoms at any one time. Furthermore, although not specific to schizophrenia, negative symptoms do appear to be more common among schizophrenic patients than among other diagnostic groups (for a review of these data, see Pogue-Geile and Zubin 1988). As the pathologic correlates of negative symptoms are reviewed elsewhere in this volume (see Chapters 5–12), we will focus here on what the presence of the negative syndrome might mean with respect to delineating etiologically heterogeneous subtypes of schizophrenia. Since genetic influences are currently the most certain etiologic agents in schizophrenia, the best evidence on this point comes from twin and family studies that have also incorporated measures of negative symptoms. These investigations have yielded the following information.

First are studies of homotypia, or the degree of similarity for negative symptoms shown by pairs of relatives who are concordant for schizophrenia. Two studies of the homotypia of negative symptoms in schizophrenia have been reported, both using Gottesman and Shields's (1972) Maudsley twin sample, although with different ratings of negative symptoms. Berenbaum et al. (1987) reported a significant correlation (.74) for ratings of anhedonia among nine monozygotic (MZ) twins concordant for schizophrenia. McGuffin et al. (1987) similarly found a high degree of homotypia for ratings of Crow's Type I-Type II dichotomy for both 15 concordant MZ (73% similar) and 4 concordant dizygotic (DZ) (75% similar) twin pairs. These data suggest that there is some tendency (although not complete) for schizophrenic patients with or without negative symptoms to "breed true" in both MZ twins and in first-degree relatives. Although based on small sample sizes, such homotypia could arise among the MZ twins (who share 100% of their genes and many environmental experiences) from at least the following three potential sources.

1. The etiology (due to shared genes or shared experiences) of schizophrenic patients with negative symptoms could differ qualitatively from those without negative symptoms (correlated specific influence hypothesis).
2. The etiology of schizophrenic patients with negative symptoms could differ quantitatively from those without negative symptoms (multiple-threshold hypothesis).
3. Schizophrenic patients with negative symptoms could differ from others on independent characteristics that are relevant to negative symptoms, but not to schizophrenia (independent influence hypothesis).

Although of necessity based on very few pairs, the high degree of homotypia shown by concordant DZ twins argues against the third possibility that negative symptoms are due to genetic factors unrelated to risk for schizophrenia. Since DZ twins share on average only 50% of their genes, any genes not directly contributing to the risk for schizophrenia would generally be shared only 50% between concordant DZ twins. However, these DZ data remain consistent with an independent effect due to shared family experiences. Further study of concordant siblings and DZ twins are needed to clarify this crucial issue. Overall, the homotypia evidence to date, although extremely tentative due to small sample sizes, is consistent with an etiologic difference of some nature (either qualitative or quantitative) between schizophrenic patients with negative symptoms and those without. The evidence against this MZ similarity being merely due to some independent influence that is not etiologically relevant to schizophrenia, however, is extremely slim (i.e., high homotypia among concordant DZ twins). In any case, negative symptoms seem to show some degree of familiality.

A second group of studies has investigated the correlations in negative symptoms for MZ and DZ twins without regard to their concordance for schizophrenia. Such analyses bear on the degree to which different familial influences are important for negative symptoms. Dworkin and Lenzenweger (1984) reported a significant MZ correlation (.26) for ratings of negative symptoms based on published case histories from previous twin studies of schizophrenia (N = 151 MZ pairs). DZ twin data were not reported. Using data from Gottesman and Shields's (1972) twin study of schizophrenia, Berenbaum et al. (1985) reported significant correlations for poverty of speech for both MZ twins (.54, n = 17 pairs) and DZ twins (.60, n = 14 pairs). This result suggests that environmental experiences shared by twins, not genetic influences, might be important determinants of poverty of speech. In contrast, these investigators found in the same sample for ratings of anhedonia that MZ correlations (.53) were significantly higher than DZ correlations (−.38) (Berenbaum et al. 1987), suggesting that genetic influences are important. Dworkin and Saczynaki (1984) reported similar findings in a small sample of normal twins. Although not uniform, these few studies are consistent with the notion that negative symptoms are to some degree familial and that some may be genetically influenced.

A third group of studies has examined the association between negative symptoms among probands and familial risk for schizophrenia in general. Such designs evaluate the multiple-threshold hypothesis that negative symptom schizophrenia may be a quantitatively more, or less, genetically severe form than non-negative symptom schizophrenia. Several studies have investigated this question among MZ twin pairs. In their analysis of published twin case vignettes, Dworkin and Lenzenweger (1984) found a somewhat increased concordance for schizophrenia in general among the MZ twins of schizophrenic probands with negative symptoms (48/92 pairs, 52%) compared to those without (21/59, 36%). This trend was significant in two (or three, depending on the analysis) of the five samples evaluated. McGuffin et al. (1987) also found a nonsignificant trend in this direction for MZ twins (64% versus 53% concordance for twins of negative symptom versus non-negative symptom probands). Berenbaum et al. (1987) found that anhedonia in MZ twin probands was associated with increased nonschizophrenic diagnoses in the co-twins, but not with diagnoses of schizophrenia.

These studies of proband negative symptomatology and MZ twin schizophrenia offer some tentative support for the notion that negative symptom schizophrenia may represent a slightly more genetically severe form of the disorder, an observation strengthened by Gottesman's (1968) early findings on clinical severity, although the results do not suggest a dramatic effect, even if one is present. Given such few data, it certainly could also be that negative symptoms merely reflect some independent influence and do not mark a more genetically severe form of schizophrenia. It is also possible, although unlikely, that negative symptom schizophrenia may identify a qualitatively distinct genetic form of schizophrenia that has approximately the same familial risk pattern as non-negative symptom schizophrenia. In any case, these MZ twin data do not support the notion that negative symptom schizophrenia represents a less genetically determined form of disorder.

Several studies have also examined this question among non-MZ twin relatives. Such investigations are statistically less powerful than are studies with MZ twins. Compared with the MZ twin results, McGuffin et al. (1987) found that DZ twins of negative symptom schizophrenic probands showed a trend toward having less schizophrenia (0/11, 0%) than did the twins of non-negative symptom probands (4/21, 19%). Similarly, Kay et al. (1986c) reported that negative symptoms in probands are associated with decreased familial risk for major mental illness (not schizophrenia specifically) if assessed during the inpatient phase, but with increased risk for disorder if the probands are chronic patients. All other such studies employing nuclear families, however, have found no significant association between proband negative symptoms and risk for schizophrenia in first-degree relatives (Andreasen and Olsen 1982; Johnstone et al. 1981; Owens and Johnstone 1980; Pearlson et al. 1984; Pogue-Geile and Hogarty 1987).

To some extent, these nuclear family studies contradict the tentative suggestion from the MZ twin data that negative symptom schizophrenia may represent a slightly more genetically severe form of the disorder. This may be due to the decreased statistical power of the family studies, or the fact that they all employed the family history method, which often suffers from decreased diagnostic sensitivity because relatives are not actually interviewed in person. Alternatively, of course, these studies may be correct in suggesting that negative symptoms do not mark a genetically more severe form of schizophrenia. Aside from the reports from McGuffin and colleagues and Kay and colleagues, the nuclear family studies do not offer support for the hypothesis that negative symptom schizophrenia may represent a genetically less severe form of the disorder.

Overall, the results of these twin and family studies of negative symptoms are suggestive at best with respect to the ability of negative symptoms to mark an etiologically distinct subtype of schizophrenia. Studies of homotypia suggest that negative symptoms may be important in some fashion. The multiple-threshold model receives some support from MZ twin concordance studies that hint that negative symptoms may describe a slightly more genetically severe form of schizophrenia, although nuclear family studies do not generally support this conclusion. It remains difficult, however, to rule out conclusively the simpler independent influence hypothesis arguing that negative symptoms primarily reflect independent factors, unrelated to the liability to schizophrenia. Furthermore, the findings also remain generally consistent with the correlated specific influence hypothesis that negative symptoms might delineate a qualitatively distinct genetic form of schizophrenia with approximately the same familial risk as the non-negative form. This hypothesis, although plausible, is not, however, parsimonious. These results could also be complicated by etiologic heterogeneity within the negative symptom syndrome itself. Despite these ambiguities, the evidence is relatively consistent in suggesting that negative symptoms do tend to be familial, perhaps genetically influenced, and apparently do not identify a "nongenetic" form of schizophrenia. Given the scarcity of data, however, this review must be more heuristic than definitive. It points to the importance of and the need for additional twin and family data to address more conclusively the issue of negative symptoms and etiologic heterogeneity.

CONCLUSIONS

This review has sought to clarify some of the conceptual issues surrounding syndromes and subtypes and to review evidence on negative symptoms and schizophrenia from this perspective. The conclusions reached are firmer regarding the syndrome status of negative symptoms than they are for their subtype status. It does seem clear that a core group of negative symptoms do tend to form a coherent cross-sectional syndrome among some schizophrenic patients. Similarly, it seems unlikely that a classification based on the joint cross-sectional occurrence of both positive and negative symptoms is warranted at this time. Major questions remain, however, regarding the further boundaries of the construct. What characteristics other than poverty of speech, flat affect, and psychomotor retardation should be included? As yet, there is little conclusive evidence to aid in such decisions. Further questions for study also concern the longitudinal characteristics of negative symptoms, which are so important for any attempt to use a cross-sectional negative symptom picture to elucidate etiologic subtypes. The little evidence that exists currently suggests that negative symptoms, although having some degree of persistence, are by no means permanent (for a review, see Pogue-Geile 1989).

The evidence is considerably less clear regarding the subtype status of negative symptoms in schizophrenia. The available data do not distinguish among a number of different subtype hypotheses. Specifically, although the homotypia evidence from MZ twins suggests that negative symptoms may be an important individual difference among schizophrenic patients, their origin and relevance for subtype hypotheses are unclear. Further evidence from non-MZ twin relatives is needed to determine whether negative symptoms might reflect an etiologic subtype of schizophrenia or merely the effects of some independent, nonspecific influence. Similarly, the data on the multiple-threshold hypothesis are only tentative at best. Nevertheless, what does seem somewhat clearer is that negative symptoms appear to be familial, and perhaps genetic, and that they probably do not mark a "nongenetic" subtype of schizophrenia. Despite an abundance of theorizing on the topic, it should be clear that our ignorance is considerable regarding the possible role of negative symptoms as indicators of etiologic subtypes in schizophrenia, and that more evidence of the sort suggested above is clearly required on these questions.

Chapter 4

Negative Symptom Rating Scales

Kenneth R. Silk, M.D.
Rajiv Tandon, M.D.

Chapter 4

Negative Symptom Rating Scales

Hypotheses about the positive-negative dichotomy in schizophrenia have resulted in a dramatic increase in empirical research on negative symptom schizophrenia. This volume reflects these developments. In conjunction with this increasing interest, the number of scales proposed to rate or identify negative symptoms has proliferated. Researchers now have at their disposal approximately a dozen scales to identify, quantify, or measure change in what has been called negative symptom schizophrenia (Andreasen and Olsen 1982), the deficit form of schizophrenia (Carpenter et al. 1988), or Type II schizophrenia (Crow 1985).

Although used interchangeably at times, these three terms are certainly not synonymous. Rating scales developed by different groups of researchers reflect the particular diagnostic slant that each research center gives to the negative symptom question. These biases are expressed in the choice of domain of assessment, item selection, and interpretation of observed phenomena. For example, the Schedule for Deficit Syndrome (SDS) (Kirkpatrick et al. 1989) specifically looks for enduring, chronic symptoms that are always present no matter what the current state (acuity, depression) of the patient. Furthermore, this instrument is designed to identify (diagnose) patients with the "deficit syndrome," rather than rate the severity of negative symptoms. The Scale for the Assessment of Negative Symptoms (SANS) (Andreasen 1982), on the other hand, measures change in negative symptoms, and thus, by definition, would be quite different from the SDS on many dimensions.

Further, it must be emphasized than none of the prevailing concepts of negative symptoms has been proven to have construct

Supported in part by National Alliance for Research in Schizophrenia and Affective Disorders (NARSAD) Fellowship Extension Award (R.T.) and the Scottish Rite Schizophrenia Research Program (R.T.).

validity. Attempts have been made to evaluate construct validity by examining internal consistency of scale items and by showing how these items cluster or factor together among themselves but do not cluster together with positive symptoms. Although these statistical studies support the idea that the combination of the specific items on that scale define "some" construct, they do not provide validation of a "negative symptom" construct (Sommers 1985; Thiemann et al. 1987). Additionally, akinesia, depression, and other phenomena observed in schizophrenic patients overlap with negative symptoms and are difficult to "tease apart" using available instruments. To establish construct validity, we would need to discover how negative symptom patients differ from other patient groups (including those with positive symptom schizophrenia) on a number of independent measures, relating to genetics, biology, psychology, pathophysiology, course, treatment, and outcome variables (Bartko and Carpenter 1976; Walker 1987; Zubin 1985). Of course, we cannot begin to test construct validity without defining the cohort to be tested, and thus we need clear, reliable, and accurate rating scales. That is the focus of this chapter.

The question of which rating scale to choose is not inconsequential. All scales reflect a particular theoretical approach to negative symptoms; thus every scale has a built-in theoretical bias. The anchor points used and the choices that raters are trained to make are determined by the theoretical viewpoint of the project's primary investigators. The scale thus becomes "the operational definition of the theoretical construct" (Sommers 1985). In view of this fact, the "match" between the biases of the rating instrument, rater, and purpose of the rating takes on paramount importance.

In this chapter, we will review the scales most commonly used to identify patients and to measure change in patients with negative symptom schizophrenia. After reviewing those instruments most frequently employed to rate negative symptoms, we will compare them in terms of their major properties (Table 4-1) and symptoms assessed (Table 4-2).

SELF-RATED INSTRUMENTS

In contrast to other diagnostic groups, there are few self-rated instruments for assessing negative symptoms. Recently, however, two negative-symptom self-rating scales have been developed: the Subjective Experience of Deficits in Schizophrenia (SEDS) (Liddle and Barnes 1988) and the Subjective Deficit Syndrome Scale (SDSS) (Bitter et al. 1989; Jaeger et al. 1990).

Table 4-1. Characteristics of negative symptom scales

Characteristic	Scales											
	SANS	PANSS	SDS	KMS	NSRS	LFM	EBS	BPRS	WING	P-G	PEARL	NSA
Type of interview	NS	U-SS-P	U-SS-P	NS	SS	NS	NS	SS	SS-P	NS	NS	SS
Negative symptom items (N)	5/30	7	6	4	10	19	16	3	4	3	6	27
Interrater reliability established	Y	Y	Y	Y	Y	Y	Y	Y	Y	N	N	Y
Test-retest reliability established	N	Y	N	N	N	N	N	Y	N	N	N	N
Ability to measure change	Y	Y	N	Y	Y	Y	Y	Y	Y	Y	Y	Y
Anchor points (N)	6	7	4	5	7	3/2	3	7	5	3	5	6
Well-defined anchor points	Y	Y	Y	Y	Y	N	N	Y	Y	N	Y	Y
Approximate time to give interview (minutes)	30	30–50	NS	5	15	10	10	20	20–30	5	10	NS

Note. NS = not specified. U = unstructured. SS = semistructured. P = probe. SANS = Scale for the Assessment of Negative Symptoms. PANSS = The Positive and Negative Syndrome Scale. SDS = Schedule for the Deficit Syndrome. KMS = Krawiecka-Manchester Scale. NSRS = Negative Symptom Rating Scale. LFM = Lewine, Fogg, Meltzer Scale. EBS = Scale for Emotional Blunting. BPRS = Brief Psychiatric Rating Scale. WING = Wing Scale. P-G = Pogue-Geile Scale. PEARL = Pearlson Scale. NSA = Negative Symptom Assessment.

Table 4-2. Negative symptoms in negative symptom rating scales

Symptoms by category	Scales											
	SANS	PANSS	SDS	KMS	NSRS	LFM	EBS	BPRS	WING	P-G	PEARL	NSA
Appearance/behavior												
Slow or restricted movement	X			X	X	X		X		X		X
Expressionless face	X						X					X
Fatigue	X					X						
Poor grooming	X				X	X					X	X
Affect												
Affective flattening	X	X	X	X	X	X	X	X		X	X	X
Inappropriate affect	X			X		X						
Anhedonia	X	X	X			X	X		X			
Indifference/apathy	X	X					X	X	X			X
Shallow mood							X				X	X
Speech												
Poverty of speech	X	X	X	X	X	X	X		X	X	X	X
Poverty of content of speech	X					X						X
Incoherence of speech				X		X			X			X
Monotonous voice	X						X					X

	SANS	SDS	KMS	BPRS	EBS	LFM	NSA	P-G
Social interpersonal								
Poor rapport	X	X	X			X	X	X
Asociality	X	X	X				X	X
Lack of social grace			X					
Decreased sexual interest	X	X	X	X			X	X
Emotional withdrawal	X	X	X	X		X		
Absence of friends	X					X		
Attention/cognition								
Stereotypic thinking	X		X				X	X
Memory impairment					X			
Attentional impairment	X				X			
Disorientation					X			
Loose associations					X			
Blocking	X							X

Note. SANS = Scale for the Assessment of Negative Symptoms. PANSS = The Positive and Negative Syndrome Scale. SDS = Schedule for the Deficit Syndrome. KMS = Krawiecka-Manchester Scale. NSRS = Negative Symptom Rating Scale. LFM = Lewine, Fogg, Meltzer Scale. EBS = Scale for Emotional Blunting. BPRS = Brief Psychiatric Rating Scale. WING = Wing Scale. P-G = Pogue-Geile Scale. PEARL = Pearlson Scale. NSA = Negative Syndrome Assessment.

Subjective Experience of Deficits in Schizophrenia

The SEDS was developed by Liddle and Barnes (1988) and consists of 21 items arranged in six groups: abnormal thinking and concentration, disturbance of affect, impaired will and decreased energy, disturbance of perception, intolerance of stress, and disturbance of voluntary movement. Ratings are based on patients' descriptions of own behavior and examples of how abnormal experiences interfere with daily activities.

Subjective Deficit Syndrome Scale

The SDSS is based on the experimental subscale of the Subclinical Symptoms Scale (Petho and Bitter 1985) and was adapted and modified for administration to an American population (Bitter et al. 1989; Jaeger et al. 1990). The SDSS consists of 19 items that constitute subjective complaints and is based exclusively on the patient's self-report.

Additionally, the SANS has items that rate the patient's subjective evaluation of each of the five symptom complexes (Andreasen 1982). These self-rated measures have not been widely employed, and their validity-utility is essentially untested. As self-rated scales develop, it will be informative to observe how schizophrenic patients with peculiar understandings of the world and with negative symptoms of apathy or diminished sense of purpose, attend, respond, and fill out self-assessment forms that explore negative symptoms.

OBSERVER-RATED INSTRUMENTS

Some observer-rated measures involve derivations from scales used to rate a wide range of symptomatology. Examples include the Brief Psychiatric Rating Scale (BPRS) (Overall and Gorham 1962) and the Krawiecka-Manchester Scale (KMS) (Krawiecka et al. 1977). Others, such as the SANS and the Positive and Negative Syndrome Scale (PANSS) (Kay et al. 1987a, 1987b), were specifically developed to rate negative symptoms. Most rely on and are derived from scales that predated them in the psychiatric literature. There is considerable variation in their breadth, scope, and the specific items selected. Although flat affect, emotional withdrawal, and alogia are included in most scales, there is less agreement about other items. Additionally, some items, such as loosening of association and inappropriate affect, are considered negative symptoms in some scales, but positive symptoms in others. Finally, there is no consistent definition of any of the individual symptoms in these scales, leading to problems with interrater reliability (de Leon et al. 1989).

REVIEW OF SCALES

Scale for the Assessment of Negative Symptoms

The SANS is probably the scale used most frequently in negative symptom schizophrenia research. It is an enlargement of the Affective Flattening Scale (Andreasen 1979) and consists of 30 items that lead to scores in five symptom complexes: alogia, affective flattening, avolition-apathy, anhedonia-asociality, and attentional impairment. In the scoring manual, there are clear and detailed definitions for each of the items. Each item is scored on a 6-point scale ranging from 0 (no complaints or no evidence) to 5 (severe). The five symptom complexes or global symptoms were chosen by Andreasen empirically, based on her "12 years' experience in evaluating, treating, and following many schizophrenic patients in a single setting" (Andreasen 1982, p. 785). In addition to the five symptom complex scores, one can determine a summary score, which sums the five global symptom complex scores, and a composite score, which sums each of the 30 items. In the composite score, one can chose to count or not to count the patient's subjective ratings of each of the five symptom complexes. There is no defined time frame over which the rated symptom or item is assessed; Andreasen suggested 1 month. There is no particular reason stated for choosing this time frame except that the author developed the instrument not only to rate negative symptoms, but also to be able to rate the change in those symptoms over time, particularly with respect to treatment. No particular interview strategy is outlined for the rater to follow, although the rater is encouraged to review hospital records and nurses' notes and to discuss the patient directly with nursing and other personnel on the unit before making ratings. Interrater reliabilities were as follows: individual items, .70–.92; the five symptom complex scores, .70–.88; the summary score, .84; and the composite, .92. The SANS has been translated into other languages, and interrater reliability has been replicated in the foreign-language versions (Dieterle et al. 1986; Mathai et al. 1986; Moscarelli et al. 1987; Obiols et al. 1985).

The Schedule for the Deficit Syndrome

Developed at the Maryland Psychiatric Research Center, the SDS assesses the presence or absence of the deficit syndrome of schizophrenia (Carpenter et al. 1988). The rationale for its development is discussed elsewhere (Carpenter et al., Chapter 1, this volume). It rates six negative symptoms: restricted affect, poverty of speech, diminished emotional range, diminished social drive, diminished sense of purpose, and curbing of interests. It generates a global severity and global deficit score. Based in part on the Quality of Life Scale (Heinrichs et al. 1984), which was rooted in the quality of life concept for schizophrenic patients introduced by Malm et al. (1981), it attempts to distinguish between transitory negative symptoms that could be related to akinesia, dysphoria, recent (exacerbation of) psychosis, understimulating environment, or chronic medications (Carpenter et al. 1985) and true chronic negative symptoms, called deficit symptoms. Items are rated from 0 (normal) to 4 (severely impaired). Items are clearly described, and a set of suggested probes is provided for each item. Descriptions are provided for anchor points. Because the scale seeks to emphasize chronic deficit symptoms, the time frame over which the items are evaluated is crucial. Thus, before rating a patient, the rater must be familiar with that patient's longitudinal course of illness, including periods of relapse and relative remission. This information should be obtained from as many sources as possible. The patient should then be evaluated for the presence of deficit symptoms at baseline and during a period of clinical stability. To qualify for the deficit syndrome, a patient must 1) meet the DSM-III-R (American Psychiatric Association 1987) criteria for schizophrenia; 2) have at least two of the six deficit symptoms listed above; 3) have no indication that the deficit symptom is caused by depression, anxiety, drug effect, or environmental deprivation; and 4) have deficit symptoms that have been present for the preceding 12 months.

Interrater reliability (weighted kappa) ranged from .60 to .73 for individual items, with .72 for global severity and .73 for global deficit (Kirkpatrick et al. 1989). It should be emphasized that this scale rates the presence or absence of the deficit syndrome and is not an instrument to rate severity of negative symptoms.

The Positive and Negative Syndrome Scale

The PANSS has 30 items, 18 of which are adapted from the BPRS and 12 from the Psychopathology Rating Schedule (Singh and Kay 1975a). The development of this scale is discussed elsewhere (Kay, Chapter 2, this volume). Items included as negative are blunted affect, emotional withdrawal, poor rapport, passive-apathetic social withdrawal, difficulty in abstract reasoning, lack of spontaneity, and stereotyped thinking. Items are scored on a 7-point scale (1–7). Each anchor point is precisely described, with instructions to assign the highest applicable rating point, even if criteria for lower ratings are also met. The scale yields a positive symptom score (from 7 items), a negative symptom score (from 7 items), and a global psychopathology score from the other 16 items. In addition, one can determine a composite scale, which expresses the direction and magnitude of difference between positive and negative symptoms. The PANSS rating is based on symptoms and functioning of the previous week. Data are elicited from multiple sources, including the patient, staff, and family. The PANSS requires a 30- to 40-minute semistructured interview with the patient. The scale has good internal consistency, with alphas ranging from .62 to .70 for mean-item totals correlated with scale totals and from .64 to.84 for individual items. Test-retest reliability (Pearson r) ranges from .60 to .80, with interrater reliability .81–.88. Positive and negative composite scores were not found to be influenced by race, cultural group, chronicity of illness, depressive symptoms, sad affect, verbal intelligence, temporal attention, or perceptual motor development (Kay et al. 1986c).

Negative Symptom Rating Scale

Developed by Iager et al. (1985) at the National Institute of Mental Health, the 10-item, 7-point (0–6) Negative Symptom Rating Scale (NSRS) is conceptually derived from descriptions of defect states in the literature. Trying to avoid the redundancy found in other scales, an attempt was made to make it short, concise, and precise. According to the authors, it requires about 10 minutes to complete. It is divided into four subscales, two with two items and two with three items. The scales assess: 1) thought process through speech and judgment–decision making; 2) cognition through memory, attention, and orientation; 3) volition through grooming, motivation, and motion; and 4) affect and relatedness through emotional response and expressive relatedness. Patients are rated on their symptoms and behavior over a given period, but the period is not specified. The interview to be used is semistructured, but no other guidelines are issued except that eliciting information to score the NSRS should guide the content and direction of the interview. Information used to score should primarily come from the patient interview, and only when information from the patient is insufficient should the rater seek other sources of information (e.g., the staff). Raters are instructed to assign the highest (better functioning) score possible for a given item, even if criteria for lower ratings are also met for that item. The interrater reliability (intraclass correlation coefficient) for the total score was 0.96; for subscale scores it ranged from .78 to .98. Kappa scores for individual items ranged from .28 to .85, with only 4 of 10 items with kappa > .5. Weighted kappa was, as expected, better, with individual item scores ranging from .57 to .97. An attempt was made to address the construct validity of the scale by comparing it to four other scales: the SANS, the Emotional Blunting Scale (EBS) (Taylor and Abrams 1978), the BPRS, and the KMS. It also was compared to the Hamilton

Rating Scale for Depression (HRSD) (Hamilton 1960). The authors found high (Spearman) correlations between the NSRS and the four other scales that measure negative symptoms, but no correlation between the NSRS and the HRSD. The psychometric limitations of this scale have been detailed by Kay et al. (1986a).

The Lewine, Fogg, and Meltzer Scale

The Lewine, Fogg, and Meltzer Scale (LFMS) was developed by Lewine et al. (1983). The scale incorporates items from the Nurses' Observation Scale for Inpatient Evaluation, 30-item version (NOSIE-30) (Honigfeld et al. 1966) and the Schedule for Affective Disorders and Schizophrenia (SADS) (Endicott and Spitzer 1978). Items were broadly drawn from the prior scales based on conceptual considerations. A mathematical formula called the Rasch model was then applied to derive a "best fit" model. The result was eight NOSIE items—sits a lot, neat (-), does things (-), speaks (-), messy, sleeps a lot, is slow, clean (-)—that are rated on a 3-point scale (absent, moderate, severe), and 11 SADS items—fatigue, loss of interest, loss of sexual interest, slowed speech, slowed body movements, depressed appearance, inappropriate affect, blunted affect, loose associations, poverty of content, and incoherence—that are rated on a 2-point (present or absent) scale. Interrater reliability was .82 for the NOSIE items and .68 for the SADS negative items. The stability of the item scores over a 2-week period was quite good, particularly in the 2 weeks directly before discharge, when patient symptoms were assumed to have stabilized.

The Krawiecka-Manchester Scale

The KMS, a short set of 5-point (0–4) items developed to rate psychotic patients, was designed to be quite sensitive to change (Krawiecka et al. 1977; Vaughn and Krawiecka 1977). Test administration takes little time. The scale employs patient interviews, clinical notes, and other sources of information in scoring. Although there is no specific interview schedule, the items and anchor points are clearly defined. Four items—incoherence and irrelevance of speech, poverty of speech or muteness, flattened or incongruous affect, and psychomotor retardation—are scored on the patient's response to questions in these areas. The other four items— depression, anxiety, delusions, and hallucinations—are scored based primarily on the rater's observations, but response to rater's questions also may be utilized here. The questions asked by the rater are open ended. Interrater reliability determined by Kendall's coefficient of concordance, W, reveals interrater reliabilities in the range of .58 to

.87, with flattened or incongruous affect faring the worst. Strong correlations were found among the items of poverty of speech, flattened or incongruous affect, and psychomotor retardation (Vaughn and Krawiecka 1977). Johnstone et al. (1978b) increased the scale to nine items by dividing flattened affect and incongruous affect into two separate items. The Northwick Park investigators (e.g., Crow, Johnstone) have exclusively utilized this scale in their studies of negative symptoms.

Pearlson Scale

Pearlson et al. (1984) used two items as defined in the KMS—poverty of speech and emotional flattening—and added four others—apathy, poor personal hygiene, absence of friends, and asexuality—to define their negative-symptom construct. No psychometric properties were described.

Emotional Blunting Scale

The EBS was developed by reviewing the literature from Pinel's era to 1978 to determine clinical descriptions of emotional blunting. This construct is all that the scale measures. Descriptive phrases are listed under the headings of affect, thought content, and behavior. These are reduced to 16 items: 4 affect, 8 behavior, and 4 thought content. Items are scored on a 3-point scale (0–2). Anchor points are not defined beyond 0 = absent, 1 = slight or doubtful, 2 = clearly present. There is no specific interview to score the 16 statements. Weighted kappas for the 16 individual items ranged from .32 to .76, with 12 of the 16 achieving a weighted kappa of > .5 and 8 of the 16 a weighted kappa > .6. Predictive validity was assessed by comparing total scores with response to treatment; subjects with higher blunting scores showed a poorer response to treatment.

Brief Psychiatric Rating Scale

The BPRS, (Overall and Gorham 1962; Overall 1974), developed specifically to measure change, was derived from two previous scales, the Multidimensional Scale for Rating Psychiatric Patients (Lorr et al. 1953) and the Inpatient Multidimensional Psychiatric Scale (Lorr et al. 1960). The BPRS is based on a 7-point scale (1–7) with each of the 16 (or 18, depending on the version) items defined. The anchor points were not defined in the original version, although some specifications have been provided in the newer versions. A semistruc-tured interview format was suggested for the BPRS. It was designed to take 18 minutes, with the first 3 minutes used to establish connec-tion and a rapport, the next 10 minutes devoted to nondirective interaction, and the last 5 minutes to direct questioning. There have been at least 22 reports supporting the reliability of the scale, particularly as an instrument for measuring change (Hedlund and Vieweg 1980). Various combinations of items (including emotional withdrawal, motor retardation, blunted affect, mannerisms and posturing, conceptual disorganization, and uncooperativeness) have been utilized to measure negative symptoms, although usually only the first three (emotional withdrawal, motor retardation, and blunted affect), constituting the 'ANER' factor, are used.

Wing Scale

Developed at Maudsley Hospital by J. K. Wing (1961), the Wing Scale was meant to assess and classify patients with chronic schizophrenia. It is not an instrument designed to measure change. Its purpose is to subclassify patients with chronic schizophrenia according to the patient's rating on four dimensions: flatness of affect, poverty of speech, incoherence of speech, and coherently expressed delusions. There is also a fifth factor, a kind of global factor related to severity of illness. A 5-point scale (1–5) is used, with anchor points partially defined. Assessment is done with a semistructured interview. The first 10 minutes are devoted to establishing rapport and asking neutral questions of the patient, the next 10–20 minutes to asking more direct questions about specific symptoms. Correlation coefficients for interrater reliability among trained raters ranged from .78 to .93 for the four factors.

Pogue-Geile and Harrow Scale

Pogue-Geile and Harrow (1984) derived a negative symptom scale from the Behavior Rating Schedule of the Psychiatric Assessment Interview (Carpenter et al. 1976), which in turn is a modification by Strauss and Carpenter (1974) of the eighth edition of the Present State Examination (World Health Organization 1974). Individual items—flat affect, poverty of speech, and psychomotor retardation—were rated on a 3-point scale (0–2), with a total score obtained from the sum of these items.

The Negative Symptom Assessment

The Negative Symptom Assessment (NSA) (Alphs et al. 1989) was developed at the Maryland Psychiatric Research Center, where the SDS was also developed. The SDS, as noted above, is a diagnostic instrument to assess the presence or absence of the deficit syndrome and does not assess negative symptom severity. The NSA, on the other hand, is designed to measure severity of negative symptoms. The authors' concept of negative symptoms is viewed ". . . as those behavioral and social abilities present in normal persons that are often lacking in individuals with schizophrenia" (Alphs et al. 1989, p. 159). The NSA has 27 items and 1 global item. Items are scored on a 6-point scale, with anchor points defined from absent (1) to severe (6). Subjects are given the highest possible scores, and scoring is based primarily on what the rater observes and what the patient reports during a semistructured interview as well as what the patient reports about his or her behavior over the previous week. Six categories of items were established a priori: communication, affect-emotion, social activity, interests, cognition, and psychomotor activity. Principal components analysis of items led to seven factors: affect-emotion, external involvement, retardation, personal presentation, thinking, interpersonal interest, and blocking. Interrater reliability (intraclass coefficient) for the NSA was .85. Construct validity was determined by principal components analysis with varimax rotation from 100 subjects and led to the seven factors listed above, each with eigenvalues > 1. There was a high correlation between the NSA total scores, the SANS total scores, and the BPRS 'ANER' scores.

DISCUSSION

As evident, there is considerable variation in the conceptualization of negative symptoms and the assessment techniques utilized by the various instruments. Although all these scales attempt to measure some theoretical construct of negative symptoms (Lewine and Sommers 1985), the question of validity of the scales and of the construct remains (Sommers 1985; Thiemann et al. 1987). Because of the variation in definitions, it is difficult to assess whether an instrument used in a particular study actually measures what it purports to measure. Additionally, although interrater reliability is often reported by the group of researchers who developed the instrument, other researchers who use the instrument in other locations often do not achieve comparable interrater reliability. Even if they do, there is no way of knowing whether the interrater reliability of the new group is in any way related to the interrater reliability of the original developers of the instrument: "the discriminations raters are taught to make when assessment instruments are ambiguous are determined by the theoretical viewpoint of the individual investigator" (Sommers 1985, p. 367). Thus the generalizability of a given study becomes questionable.

Most scales do not specify who should rate the patient. Often it is the least clinically sophisticated member of a research team, the research assistant or associate, who is charged with rating the patient.

Patients with negative symptom schizophrenia have a tendency to be withdrawn, unmotivated, and passive. It might be more appropriate to have the most experienced and sophisticated clinicians complete the rating (Sommers 1985). Further, ratings by a research psychiatrist, no matter how sophisticated he or she may be, may differ from those made by the patient's primary clinician, who has established some ongoing relationship, no matter how tenuous, with the patient and who may be trusted much more than anyone else on the treatment or research team.

None of the scales has a specifically designed structured interview attached to it. Some interviews are open ended, some semistructured, and some simple and direct to probe for the particular symptom being rated. There are probably many advantages to using a semistructured interview that allow for individual patient differences and permit the rater to probe and question, particularly when dealing with patients who are vague and unmotivated. Nonetheless, the semistructured format encourages rater bias. Further, if anchor points are not clearly defined, what may be "severe" to one rater may be only "moderate" to another.

Every one of these measures provides users with information, but it is the task of the researcher to select carefully the most appropriate instrument for a study. Although great attention is paid to the formulation of the overall methodology of a study, less rigor may be applied when selecting instruments of assessment. We can choose imprecise instruments or use them improperly to measure phenomena they were not designed to measure. The instruments may have been designed for use on a more narrowly defined group of patients than the ones being studied. Inconsistency among observers and raters because of training or theoretical bias can also be a major source of error (Thiemann et al. 1987).

The use of internal consistency as a measure of validity should be viewed with caution. Internal consistency may reflect the "tightness" of the theoretical construct of the scale, or it may simply mean that the items of the scale are measuring different aspects of the same phenomenon. Additionally, the possibility exists that a subject who scores high on any one item of a particular scale will automatically score high on every other item in that scale ("the halo effect"). The rater will come to assume that the other items are present as soon as the first item is found to be present, and then internal theoretical bias is reported as internal consistency.

The multiplicity of definitions and instruments means that researchers who select any one instrument run the risk of missing crucial information. Researchers who select a scale based on a narrow definition may omit informative items, whereas those that select a broad definition confront the problem of diluting the concept and blurring its demarcation from other phenomena. Researchers attempting to use multiple instruments must expend considerable time and money. They also risk compromising the interpretability of their findings because 1) the different scales may yield inconsistent or conflicting findings, and 2) there is a greater likelihood of Type I error related to an increase in the number of statistical tests, leading to significant findings by chance alone (Thiemann et al. 1987).

This discussion is not meant to dissuade people from using available rating instruments. All scales have their advantages and disadvantages, many of which are determined not by the instrument itself but by the purposes for which the instrument is being used. Careful consideration of all the instruments ideally should lead to selection of the best method of assessment for a particular study. Because of the limitations described above, the use of multiple raters and possibly of multiple instruments is to be encouraged. The psychometric properties of the instrument(s) must be reevaluated by the investigators. Knowledge beforehand of the weaknesses and biases of the instrument will mitigate against too many surprises during data analysis and help prevent not only Type I error, but perhaps, more importantly, Type II error as well.

Although the issues discussed in this chapter suggest methodological limitations in the generalization of findings of the various studies on negative symptoms and indicate variation in the conceptualization of the negative symptom construct, it should not be implied that the construct itself is not useful or is invalid. On the contrary, the burgeoning literature and large number of rating scales attest to the perceived importance of the concept, despite the difficulty in defining it. Although a consensus on the definition and measurement of negative symptoms would be useful, investigators face the tension (as described by Popper 1963) between wanting to be quite sure of what we are talking about and wanting to get on with the job of finding out about it. The first chapters in this volume (including this one) have been concerned with the first issue; subsequent chapters are concerned with the latter. An improved conceptualization of negative symptoms will clearly result from a combination of these strategies.

Biochemical Hypotheses

Chapter 5

Prefrontal Dopamine and Defect Symptoms in Schizophrenia

Karen Faith Berman, M.D.
Daniel R. Weinberger, M.D.

Chapter 5

Prefrontal Dopamine and Defect Symptoms in Schizophrenia

The dopamine hypothesis has been one of the cornerstones of schizophrenia research and treatment for many years (Meltzer and Stahl 1976). In brief, this theory holds that schizophrenia results, at least in part, from a functional overactivity or overabundance of dopamine in the brain. Support for the dopamine hypothesis arose from the clinical observations that dopamimetic agents can cause psychosis (Angrist et al. 1974) and that agents that block the action of dopamine at its receptors—classically the D_2 subtype of receptors—ameliorate positive symptoms of schizophrenia such as hallucinations and delusions (Carlsson 1978).

It is well accepted, however, that neuroleptics do not ameliorate the negative, or defect, symptoms of schizophrenia, such as amotivation and anhedonia, and that dopamimetics given acutely do not cause them. Thus the dopamine hypothesis, at least as classically stated, may not be entirely applicable to negative symptoms. This is not to say that the dopamine system does not have an important role in the pathogenesis of negative symptoms. On the contrary, we suggest in this chapter that a relative deficiency of dopamine in certain crucial brain areas and an imbalance among the various components of the dopamine system may be key pathogenic features of negative symptoms.

Since this suggestion constitutes a considerable departure from the original dopamine hypothesis, we must reconcile it with the observations on which that theory was founded. Resolution of these seemingly disparate formulations may lie in the growing body of new information about dopamine in the brain. This new knowledge has been derived from several different but complementary approaches to research in neuroscience. For example, recent studies of the non-human primate (Brozowski et al. 1979) (which compared with the rat is a much better, although still imperfect, model for the human dopamine system) have elucidated the importance of dopamine in certain cognitive processes and refined our knowledge of the anatomy of the primate dopamine system. Concurrently, the development of drugs that are selectively active at the several pharmacologically and biochemically distinct dopamine receptor subtypes has allowed neuropharmacologic studies in both rodents and primates that have clarified the roles of these receptor subtypes. Finally, the emergence of in vivo imaging techniques has allowed direct assessment of brain neurochemistry and physiology in the living, working human brain. With these new data and tools, we can begin to delineate the neurobiology of defect symptoms.

PRECLINICAL STUDIES OF BRAIN DOPAMINE

Two Dopamine Receptor Subtypes

Dopamine, like other neurotransmitters, is synthesized in neurons and stored in synaptic vesicles. If a dopaminergic neuron is activated, dopamine is released into the synapse, where it meets one of three fates: it may be inactivated or metabolized to homovanillic acid (HVA), it may be removed from the synapse through reuptake by the neuron that produced it, or it may become bound to a receptor site on another neuron. These receptor sites are protein complexes within the plasma membrane of each neuron. There are two pharmacologically and functionally distinct subtypes of dopamine receptors: D_1 and D_2 (Burt et al. 1976). The D_1 receptors stimulate adenylate cyclase activity, whereas the D_2 receptors inhibit this enzymic second messenger.

Although neuroleptics can block both D_1 and D_2 receptors, most studies of the action of neuroleptics on the dopamine system have focused on the D_2 subtype, possibly because a high correlation between the clinical doses of the various neuroleptic drugs and their affinity at the D_2 receptor has been demonstrated (Creese et al. 1976; Seeman et al. 1976). The relationship with D_1 receptors, however, remains unclear. In fact, many butyrophenones and substituted benzamide neuroleptics are only weakly active at the D_1 receptor. Nevertheless, with the recent availability of agents that are selective for the D_1 receptor, it has become clear that there are important interactions between the D_1 and D_2 receptors and that the D_1 receptors, too, are behaviorally important (Braun et al. 1986).

The majority of dopamine receptor studies in schizophrenia have also focused on the D_2 system. The most consistent postmortem finding in schizophrenia is perhaps that of increased D_2 receptors in autopsied basal ganglia and limbic system (for a review, see Kleinman et al. 1988). However, since the administration of neuroleptic medications has been shown to increase the number of dopamine receptors in animals, and since most patients with schizophrenia would have received neuroleptics by the time they come to autopsy, it has not been possible to exclude the possibility that the increased D_2 receptors in schizophrenic brains may simply reflect previous treatment.

Recent investigations using positron emission tomography (PET) to measure D_2 receptors in vivo have attempted to address this methodological problem by studying patients with schizophrenia who have never been treated with neuroleptics. Although one such study found that the density of D_2 receptors was increased in the basal ganglia of schizophrenic patients (Wong et al. 1986), another group of investigators was not able to confirm this finding (Farde et al. 1987, 1990). The fact that the two groups of investigators used different D_2 ligands and different mathematical models to determine receptor density may explain the apparent inconsistency. Further studies will be necessary to clarify this important question.

In contrast to the above-mentioned evidence that there may be a relative overabundance of D_2 receptors in schizophrenia, few studies of the D_1 receptor have been published. However, Hess et al. (1987) measured both D_1 and D_2 receptors in postmortem caudate nuclei of patients with schizophrenia and normal controls. They found that while there was an increase in D_2 receptors in the patients, the number of D_1 receptors was decreased. If this finding is replicated, it may point the way toward new approaches for treatment, such as selective D_1 agonists and partial agonists. PET studies of D_1 receptors in patients have not yet been reported. Such measurements in living subjects would allow concurrent assessment of neuroreceptor status and clinical phenomena, which may help to clarify the role of the D_1 system in such clinical features as negative symptoms.

Anatomy of the Primate Dopamine System

The cell bodies in which the dopamine system originates are located primarily in the substantia nigra and in the ventral tegmental area. Several anatomically distinct (although interrelated) dopamine systems arise from these cells. A nigrostriatal system, a mesolimbic system, and a mesocortical system are usually described. The nigrostriatal system projects to the caudate, putamen, and globus pallidus; the mesolimbic system projects to limbic regions, including hypothalamus, hippocampus, amygdala, and nucleus accumbens; and the mesocortical system projects to the cortex, particularly prefrontal cortex.

There have been relatively few studies comparing D_1 and D_2 receptor populations in various brain regions. Preliminary evidence suggests that in the primate brain both D_1 and D_2 receptors are located subcortically. The cortical dopamine system, however, may consist mainly of D_1 receptors. In vivo imaging of receptors with ligands specific to the D_1 and D_2 receptor types will help to delineate further the anatomy of the dopamine system in the human brain.

Although the precise pathways have yet to be thoroughly traced, it is clear that in the normal brain there are complex feedback circuits between the prefrontal cortical and subcortical dopamine systems. It appears, for example, that mesocortical dopamine neurons affect prefrontal cortical neurons that in turn exert feedback control over mesolimbic activity (Thierry et al. 1984). Pycock et al. (1980) demonstrated in the rat that a disruption of this system at the level of the prefrontal cortex can cause the "brakes" to be taken off the subcortical dopamine system, resulting in a functional hyperactivity of basal ganglia and limbic dopamine. This scenario is one by which a brain could simultaneously have too much dopamine subcortically (consistent with the classical dopamine hypothesis) and too little dopamine cortically.

A Model for Conceptualizing Schizophrenia

Weinberger (1987) proposed that a dysregulation of the dopamine systems similar to that described above may occur in the brains of patients with schizophrenia (Figure 5-1). The putative hypofunction of the prefrontal dopamine system could provide a possible neurobiologic mechanism for negative symptoms; the increased subcortical dopamine activity might account for positive symptoms and movement disorder. The combination of positive and negative symptoms common in schizophrenia could result from reduced prefrontal dopamine function, leading to relative hyperactivity of subcortical dopamine, which would normally be modulated by the prefrontal system. Of course, this formulation likely is an over-simplification, and the involvement of cortical dopamine itself may be an epiphenomenon. It may be important only to have prefrontal dysfunction and loss of cortical feedback. Such a phenomenon has actually been demonstrated in the rat (Jaskiw et al., unpublished observations).

We now have the means to explore experimentally this interesting possibility, although it has not been proven in the human brain. The observations presented above make clear that it is no longer sufficient to talk simplistically about "too much" or "too little" dopamine in the brain. Tools such as in vivo imaging of neuroreceptors, selective D_1 and D_2 agonists and antagonists, and careful postmortem methods will be crucial in determining where alterations in brain dopamine function occur, whether the changes are pre- or postsynaptic, and how the various components of the brain's dopamine system may interact to produce dysfunction.

CLINICAL AND NEUROBIOLOGIC CORRELATES

Cerebrospinal Fluid Metabolites and Negative Symptoms

The first question that must be asked in the present context is whether there is any evidence to support the notion of a relative deficit of dopamine function in schizophrenia and in negative symptoms. The study of Hess et al. (1987) demonstrating decreased D_1 receptors in

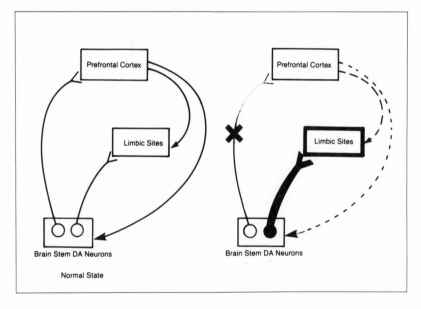

Figure 5-1. Schematized interactions between mesolimbic and mesocortical dopamine systems in normal state (*left*) and after selective lesioning of dopamine input to prefrontal cortex (*right*), based on work of Pycock et al. 1980. *Broken line* indicates that the specific effect of lesion on corticolimbic feedback (e.g., decreased inhibition or increased excitation) is unknown. DA = dopamine. (Adapted from Weinberger 1987.)

postmortem human brain supports this notion. Other literature addressing this question is somewhat inconsistent, but several studies of the levels of neurotransmitter metabolites support this theory. Davidson and Davis (1988) found lower plasma HVA levels in schizophrenic patients than in normal controls. Karoum et al. (1987) reported that 24-hour urinary excretion of dopamine and its metabolites was reduced in patients.

In 1974, Bowers and Rozitis showed that patients with schizophrenia had lower cerebrospinal fluid (CSF) levels of the dopamine metabolite HVA than did patients with affective disorder. Moreover, the poor-prognosis, "burnt out" patients had lower HVA levels than did those with a better prognosis. More recently, Lindstrom (1985) demonstrated that, while levels of the serotonergic marker 5-hydroxyindolacetic acid were normal in schizophrenia, CSF HVA levels were decreased, and the amount of the decrease correlated with the severity and number of defect symptoms. Thus there is evidence to suggest that, at least in some patients, there may be decreased dopamine and that this decrease is related to negative symptoms.

Prefrontal Cortex and Negative Symptoms

The prefrontal cortex may also play a role in negative symptoms. The prefrontal lobe can be roughly considered as two systems: a dorsolateral system and an orbitomedial system. Studies of patients with lesions show that injury of the dorsolateral prefrontal cortex can produce a syndrome much like the negative symptoms of schizophrenia, including decreased initiative and motivation, emotional blunting, impoverished thinking, social withdrawal, lack of insight and judgment, poor personal hygiene, and impaired problem solving (Stuss and Benson 1986).

There is more direct evidence that dysfunction of dorsolateral prefrontal cortex (hypofrontality) is related to negative symptoms (in particular, impaired problem solving) and to dopaminergic function. Data demonstrating hypofrontality in schizophrenia date back to the landmark studies of Ingvar and Franzen (1974). Using the intracarotid xenon technique, they showed that while nonschizophrenic control subjects were hyperfrontal (having the highest levels of blood flow to anterior cortical areas), patients with schizophrenia were relatively hypofrontal (i.e., showing relatively decreased frontal function). Importantly, these investigations further showed that there was a correlation between the degree of hypofrontality and how autistic, deteriorated, and "burned out" the patients were. This finding has been confirmed by Volkow et al. (1987), who reported that patients with more negative symptoms showed more severe hypofrontality (i.e., lower frontal cerebral glucose metabolism as measured with PET) than did patients with fewer negative symptoms.

We and others (Berman et al. 1986, 1988; Cohen et al. 1987b; Volkow et al. 1987; Weinberger et al. 1986) have shown that hypofrontality may be behavior specific; that is, hypofunction of prefrontal cortex is consistently seen during activities that place a physiologic load on prefrontal cortex. Hypofrontality is less consistently observed during activities that are not specifically linked to prefrontal cortex, such as the resting state. For example, during a behavior that in normal subjects causes increased metabolic activity in the dorsolateral prefrontal cortex and requires that this area be intact (i.e., performance of the Wisconsin Card Sort Test [WCS (Grant and Berg 1948; Milner 1963)]), no such activation was seen in patients (Berman et al. 1986; Weinberger et al. 1986) (see Figure 5-2). We have recently replicated this finding (Weinberger et al. 1988b). In contrast, we were not able to demonstrate hypofrontality during a simple numbers matching task (Berman et al. 1986; Weinberger et al. 1986, 1988b), during attentional tasks (Berman et al. 1986), or during a difficult abstract reasoning task that is not linked to prefrontal cortex (Berman et al. 1988). Furthermore, the results of our first WCS blood flow study (Weinberger et al. 1986) suggested that a patient's success in performing the WCS may depend on the degree to which he or she shows activation of prefrontal cortex.

Prefrontal Physiology and Dopamine

In addition to its association with negative symptoms such as impaired problem solving, prefrontal activity appears to be directly linked to the level of dopaminergic function in schizophrenia. We found a relationship between CSF levels of the dopamine metabolite HVA and hyperfrontality during the WCS, but not during a simple numbers matching paradigm that does not specifically require the involvement of prefrontal cortex (Figure 5-3). Higher HVA levels correlated with higher relative prefrontal flow in the patients (Weinberger et al. 1988b). This suggests a role for dopamine in mediating this behavior-specific hypofrontality and the concomitant cognitive deficits in schizophrenia.

It is difficult to make inferences about the status of brain dopaminergic function on the basis of concentrations of metabolites in the lumbar CSF; it might seem even more problematic to draw conclusions about dopaminergic function in specific brain areas on this basis. There are now several studies in the literature that may clarify this issue. It has been traditionally assumed that CSF HVA levels primarily reflect nigrostriatal activity. A study by Ellsworth et al. (1987) in the monkey, however, does not support this view and, in fact, provides evidence linking CSF HVA levels specifically to dorsolateral prefrontal cortex. They found that CSF HVA levels did not correlate with striatal or orbitofrontal HVA concentrations, but did correlate with the levels in the dorsolateral cortex. A similar relationship between prefrontal HVA and CSF HVA in human postmortem material has also been reported (Stanley et al. 1985). If CSF HVA levels indeed mainly reflect prefrontal dopaminergic ac-

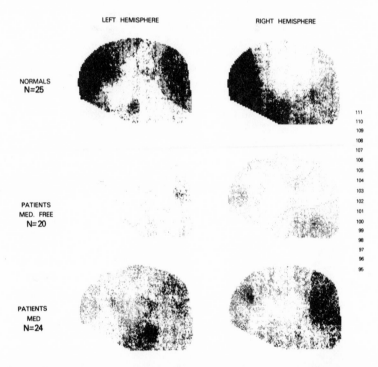

Figure 5-2. Regional cerebral blood flow (rCBF). Lateral view (with anterior pole at *left*) of left and right hemisphere percentage of change in rCBF during the Wisconsin Card Sort (WCS) compared with rCBF during a number matching control task. Data are for 25 normal control subjects (*top*), 20 medication-free patients (*middle*), and 24 neuroleptic-treated patients (*bottom*). Note that the control subjects, unlike either patient group, show striking rCBF increases (i.e., darker shades) during WCS in an area corresponding to dorsolateral prefrontal cortex. (From Berman et al. 1986 and Weinberger et al. 1986.)

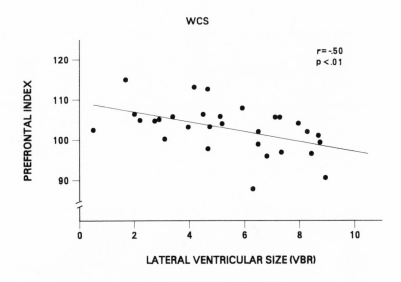

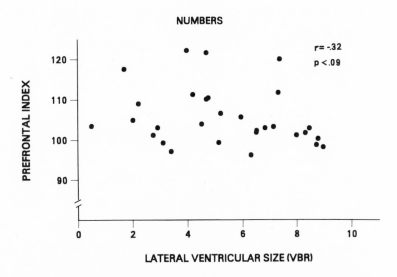

Figure 5-3. Relationship between lateral ventricular size and relative prefrontal blood flow (prefrontal index) during the Wisconsin Card Sort (*top*) ($N = 30$, $r = -.50$, $P < .01$) and the Number Matching Test (*bottom*) ($N = 30$, $r = -.32$, $P < .09$). (Adapted from Berman et al. 1987.)

tivity, the data discussed above suggest that decreased functional activity of the prefrontal dopamine system may be the neurochemical mechanism underlying behavior-specific hypofrontality.

Several other converging lines of evidence support the idea that intact dopaminergic function is necessary for adequate performance of prefrontally linked activities. Brozowski et al. (1979) demonstrated that selective regional depletion of dopamine from prefrontal cortex of rhesus monkeys caused cognitive impairment on delayed response tasks. The degree of this impairment was similar to that produced by total ablation of prefrontal cortex. Depletion of 5-hydroxytryptamine or norepinephrine did not cause cognitive deficit. Interestingly, delayed response may be the nonhuman primate equivalent of the WCS, in that it involves many of the same cognitive operations and has also been shown to depend on an intact dorsolateral prefrontal cortex.

Further evidence is found in studies of Parkinson's disease. This illness involves a loss of nigrostriatal dopamine, but, more importantly for the present discussion, it also represents a known situation of degeneration of the mesocortical dopamine pathway. Some of the cognitive and behavioral deficits of patients with Parkinson's disease that are thought to reflect diminished dopaminergic prefrontal function are phenomenologically similar to the deficit symptoms of schizophrenia (Scatton et al. 1982). In a blood flow study designed similarly to the schizophrenia studies described above (Weinberger et al. 1988a), the degree of prefrontal activation during the WCS correlated with clinical features of Parkinson's disease that are traditionally linked to dopamine deficiency (e.g., rigidity and bradykinesia), but not with severity of tremor, a sign traditionally thought to be related to the cholinergic system. We also noted a striking correlation between the degree of prefrontal activation and performance on the WCS that was in the same direction as noted in our first schizophrenia study: the more prefrontal blood flow, the fewer the perseverative errors. This observation suggests that there may be some common pathophysiologic mechanism at the cortical level in Parkinson's disease and schizophrenia.

In a related study, we explored the effects of the dopamine agonist apomorphine on regional cerebral blood flow in medication-free patients with schizophrenia during the WCS. An acute dose of apomorphine significantly reversed the WCS-related hypofrontality in the majority of patients. In a related study, amphetamine produced significant activation of the left dorso-lateral prefrontal cortex (DLPFC) during the WCS, suggesting that enhanced DLPFC monoaminergic activity may increase DLPFC metabolism and reverse "hypofrontality" in schizophrenia (Daniel et al. 1990). Chronic trials of dopaminergic agonists, both nonselective and selective for the D_1 system, both with and without agents to block the D_2 system, are currently under way.

Structural Pathology, Dopamine, and Negative Symptoms

One clue to the mechanism underlying the prefrontal cortical pathophysiology described above may lie in subcortical brain structures. We found that the degree of hypofrontality in patients was linked to a putative measure of subcortical structural pathology: enlargement of the lateral ventricles (Berman et al. 1987). The larger a patient's ventricles, the more hypofrontal he or she was. This relationship was noted when blood flow was measured during the WCS, but not during the simple numbers matching task (Figure 5-4). This pattern of a behaviorally specific correlation is remarkably similar to our results with HVA (Figure 5-3). A possible interpretation of these data is that there is a structural neuropathologic abnormality (reflected by enlargement of the lateral ventricles) in schizophrenia that disrupts dopaminergic innervation to the prefrontal cortex.

Indirect support for this concept comes from a number of studies showing a relationship between the size of the lateral ventricles and measures of dopamine function. For example, Nyback et al. (1983) reported a negative correlation between the size of the lateral ventricles and the level of HVA. Van Kammen et al. (1983) found inverse correlations between central dopamine activity (as indicated by CSF HVA and dopamine beta-hydroxylase levels) and both lateral ventricular enlargement and cortical atrophy. Losonczy et al. (1986b) also demonstrated a negative correlation between ventricular size and CSF HVA. Collectively, these studies suggest a link between large ventricles and reduced mesocortical dopamine activity.

Completing the picture of a constellation of neurobiologic features associated with negative symptoms is a possible relationship between enlargement of the lateral ventricles and the defect state. Although not all studies agree, several have found that negative symptoms are more prevalent in patients with large ventricles (Kemali et al. 1985; Pearlson et al. 1984; Williams et al. 1985) and that patients with large ventricles do not respond to treatment with dopamine blockers to the same degree as do patients with smaller ventricles (Weinberger et al. 1980a). This topic is reviewed in greater detail elsewhere (Olson et al., Chapter 9, this volume).

SUMMARY

In conclusion, we propose that some of the neurobiologic correlates

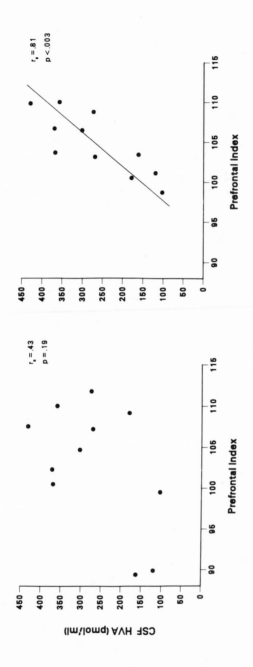

Figure 5-4. Correlations between cerebrospinal fluid (CSF) concentrations of homovanillic acid (HVA) and prefrontal index during the Number Matching Test (*left*) and the Wisconsin Card Sort (*right*) (r_s +.81, P .003). (Adapted from Weinberger et al. 1988b.)

of defect symptoms are, in fact, known. They include 1) enlargement of the lateral ventricles, 2) reduced dopamine metabolites in the CSF, and 3) metabolic hypofunction of prefrontal cortex. We would further propose that these biological markers are linked in a manner that may have meaning for the pathogenesis of schizophrenia. In addition, although it is unlikely that dysfunction of any single neurotransmitter system could account for a complex behavioral abnormality such as negative symptoms, we would also suggest that one common factor may be in these neurobiologic correlates: dopamine. This conceptual framework provides a number of hypotheses that we now have the tools to test directly.

Chapter 6

Cholinergic Excess and Negative Schizophrenic Symptoms

Rajiv Tandon, M.D.
John F. Greden, M.D.

Chapter 6

Cholinergic Excess and Negative Schizophrenic Symptoms

T he cholinergic system has intermittently been suspected of being involved in the pathophysiology of schizophrenia, but its precise role has been inadequately investigated and is still poorly understood. Some of the earliest pharmacologic interventions in schizophrenia actually involved manipulation of the cholinergic system with anticholinergic agents such as hyoscine (Kraepelin 1919) and atropine (Forrer and Miller 1958), or cholinergic stimulation with acetylcholine (Cohen et al. 1944) and arecoline (Pfeiffer and Jenney 1957). Despite these historical precedents, cholinergic mechanisms currently are considered relatively unimportant in schizophrenia and primarily discussed with regard to undesirable extrapyramidal side effects of neuroleptics. Evidence from several lines of research, however, suggests that this viewpoint warrants reconsideration. The cholinergic system may play a prominent role in schizophrenic pathophysiology; specifically, muscarinic hyperactivity may be relevant to the pathogenesis of negative schizophrenic symptoms and there may be an association between reduced cholinergic activity and positive symptoms (Tandon and Greden 1989). In this chapter, we summarize this evidence and present a model of cholinergic-dopaminergic interactions in the context of the longitudinal course of schizophrenia.

Supported in part by National Alliance for Research in Schizophrenia and Affective Disorders (NARSAD) Fellowship Extension Award (R.T.), the Scottish Rite Schizophrenia Research Program (R.T.), and NIH Grant # MO1-RR-00042 (R.T.).

99

MUSCARINIC HYPERACTIVITY AND NEGATIVE SCHIZOPHRENIC SYMPTOMS

Pharmacologic manipulation of the cholinergic system with agonists-antagonists in nonschizophrenic and schizophrenic patients, studies of biological markers of the cholinergic system in schizophrenic patients, and related experiments provide considerable evidence implicating muscarinic hyperactivity in the production of negative schizophrenic symptoms. These data have been discussed extensively by Tandon and Greden (1989) and are summarized below.

Effect of Cholinergic Stimulation in Normals

Centrally active cholinomimetic agents and cholinesterase inhibitors produce syndromes characterized by psychomotor retardation, apathy, withdrawal, lethargy, decreased energy, slowed thoughts, decreased thoughts, diminished affective responsivity, and reduced hedonic capacity (Davis et al. 1976; Greden et al. 1987; Risch et al. 1981). Although these findings have been previously hypothesized to implicate cholinergic mechanisms in depression, the similarity of this behavioral profile to the negative schizophrenic syndrome also is striking. It is possible, of course, that increased cholinergic activity may be involved in both the negative schizophrenic syndrome and certain aspects of depressive syndromes. This would account for their phenomenological similarities and for the frequent difficulty in differentiating between them in clinical settings (Sommers 1985).

Effect of Cholinergic Stimulation on Negative Schizophrenic Symptoms

Some studies have reported therapeutic benefits of cholinergic agonists and cholinesterase inhibitors in schizophrenia (Pfeiffer and Jenney 1957; Rosenthal and Bigelow 1973), but improvements have been noted principally in positive symptoms such as paranoid delusions and hallucinations. Other studies have failed to confirm such improvement in positive symptoms and have instead reported an inhibitory or "depressogenic" effect (Janowsky et al. 1973; Modestin et al. 1973; Rowntree et al. 1950). Rowntree et al. actually noted an increase in both positive and negative symptoms following chronic administration of diisopropyl fluorophosphate, an irreversible cholinesterase inhibitor. An analysis of this depressogenic effect reveals that worsening occurs chiefly in the areas of motor retardation, emotional withdrawal, anergy, and reduced speech (a profile similar to the negative syndrome). The increase in negative symptoms in schizophrenic patients following administration of cholinergic agents extends the finding of induction of negative symptoms in normal subjects following pharmacologically induced increases in cholinergic activity.

Effect of Anticholinergic Agents on Negative Symptoms

Anticholinergic agents are commonly employed in schizophrenic patients to reduce the extrapyramidal side effects that often accompany neuroleptic treatment. Although some reports suggest that such agents may interfere with the beneficial effects of neuroleptics on positive symptoms (Johnstone et al. 1983; Singh and Kay 1979b), no adverse effects on negative symptoms have been observed. Indeed, several reports have noted beneficial effects of continued antiparkinsonian medication in a sizable proportion of schizophrenic patients, and increased subjective distress, social withdrawal, and "depressive symptomatology" following withdrawal of these agents (Altamura et al. 1986; Jellinek et al. 1981; Manos et al. 1981). An open pilot study on the effects of trihexyphenidyl on negative symptoms in five chronic schizophrenic patients revealed significant improvement in four patients, particularly in the areas of affective flattening, anhedonia-asociality, and avolition-apathy (Tandon et al. 1988). Another study (Fayen et al. 1988) reported a similar improvement of negative symptoms with trihexyphenidyl in comparison to amantadine, when these agents were employed to treat neuroleptic-induced extrapyramidal side effects. We recently studied the effects of biperiden, a relatively specific M-1 antimuscarinic anticholinergic agent, on positive and negative symptoms in 15 medication-free schizophrenic inpatients (Tandon et al. 1990a). We found that while positive symptoms increased significantly ($P < .01$), there was a trend for negative symptoms to decrease ($t = 1.9$, 14 df, $P = .08$). These effects of an increase in positive symptoms and decrease in negative symptoms in drug-free schizophrenic patients following biperiden was confirmed in a larger sample (Tandon et al., in press a).

Anticholinergic Abuse in Schizophrenia

More than 30 published reports containing several hundred cases describe anticholinergic drug abuse by schizophrenic patients. Reviews of this subject (Fisch 1987; Smith 1980) have noted a high incidence of such abuse. Patients often report mood-elevating, energizing, stimulating, and socializing effects from these agents. These effects also have been observed in schizophrenic patients who were not receiving neuroleptics, suggesting that these beneficial effects are not solely attributable to relief of extrapyramidal side effects. There are virtually no comparable reports of abuse by schizophrenic patients of other prescription psychotropic drugs such as antidepressants, antipsychotics, and anxiolytics. Perhaps schizophrenic patients with prominent negative symptoms who abuse anticholinergics are indicating something about their underlying pathophysiology (possible muscarinic hyperactivity).

Polysomnographic Studies in Schizophrenia

Cholinergic mechanisms are of central importance in the tonic and phasic aspects of sleep regulation. There is particularly good evidence for cholinergic control of the onset of the first rapid-eye-movement (REM) period. Increased cholinergic activity is associated with earlier onset of the first REM period (decreased REM latency) and reduced slow-wave sleep (SWS) (Kupfer et al. 1988; Sitaram et al. 1979). Although these sleep parameters are affected by other neurotransmitter systems as well, they are significantly regulated by and serve as an indirect marker of the central muscarinic system.

Although sleep electroencephalographic studies in schizophrenia have yielded discrepant findings, a majority of studies suggest that both acute and chronic schizophrenic patients can have short REM latencies. Results of earlier studies may have been confounded by a variety of methodological problems, but five of six recent studies have confirmed the presence of shortened REM latency and increased REM density in schizophrenia (Ganguli et al. 1987; Hiatt et al. 1985; Keshavan et al. 1989c; Tandon et al. 1989a, 1989c; Zarcone et al. 1987). These findings were noted in schizophrenic patients without significant depression; furthermore, medication-free patients with schizophrenia (as defined by Spitzer et al.'s [1978] Research Diagnostic Criteria) had REM abnormalities that were indistinguishable from patients with major depressive disorder (Douglass et al. 1989; Zarcone et al. 1987).

Non-REM sleep abnormalities also have been linked to schizophrenia. SWS appears to be significantly decreased. Earlier investigations noted no association of these sleep findings with depressive symptomatology, but did not investigate their relation- ship with positive/negative or other aspects of schizophrenic symptomatology. When negative features were monitored, it was noted that decreased SWS (Ganguli et al. 1987; Tandon et al. 1989a; van Kammen et al. 1988) and short REM latency (Tandon et al. 1989a, 1989c) were both significantly correlated with negative symptoms. Since muscarinic hyperactivity is associated with both reduced SWS and REM latency, the relationship between these sleep abnormalities and negative symptoms indirectly supports the implication of increased muscarinic activity in the production of negative schizophrenic symptoms.

Neuroendocrine Studies

Since neuroendocrine measures generally are regulated by multiple neurotransmitter systems, interpreting their activity as a marker of any one particular neurotransmitter must be done cautiously. Cholinergic mechanisms are known to play a significant role in releasing corticotropin-releasing hormone and in regulating the growth hormone response to thyrotropin-releasing hormone. Negative symptom severity has been linked with postdexamethasone cortisol levels (Saffer et al. 1985; Tandon et al. 1989d) and growth hormone response to thyrotropin-releasing hormone (Keshavan et al. 1989b), particularly in the acute psychotic phase of the illness. Again, these data indirectly support the implication of increased muscarinic activity in the production of negative symptoms in this phase of the illness. These neuroendocrine findings are discussed further by Keshavan et al. (Chapter 8, this volume).

Effect of Neuroleptics on Negative Symptoms

Poor response to neuroleptics is generally considered a characteristic feature of the negative syndrome. Several studies, however, have demonstrated concomitant improvement in both positive and negative symptoms with neuroleptic treatment (Cole et al. 1966; Breier et al. 1987; Tandon et al. 1990b). This issue is discussed further by Meltzer (Chapter 14, this volume). Clozapine, an atypical neuroleptic with the most potent anticholinergic activity of the various neuroleptics (Richelson 1984; Snyder et al. 1974), is reported to be more effective than traditional neuroleptics in ameliorating negative symptoms (Kane et al. 1988). Other properties of clozapine, such as antiserotonergic (anti-5-HT$_2$), greater anti-D$_1$ activity, and relatively selective mesolimbic dopamine blockade, have been proposed as explanations of its greater efficacy in treating negative symptoms, but its potent antimuscarinic activity must be investigated as a contributing factor.

Increased Cholinergic Activity and Decreased Drive-Reduction Behavior

Muscarinic agonists consistently have been found to diminish drive reduction behavior in humans and other animals (Domino and Olds 1968). Decrease in drive reduction is closely related to anhedonia, a prominent negative symptom.

DECREASED MUSCARINIC ACTIVITY AND POSITIVE SYMPTOMS

While studies are underway to test the hypothesis that muscarinic hyperactivity may be related to negative symptoms, several authors have previously suggested that cholinergic activity actually may be decreased in schizophrenia (Davis et al. 1975; Friedhoff and Alpert 1973; Janowsky et al. 1973; Singh and Kay 1985). A number of observations are relevant.

First, general clinical experience suggests that anticholinergic drugs do not adversely affect neuroleptic efficacy, but several investigators (Johnstone et al. 1983, 1988; Singh and Kay 1979b; Singh et al. 1987) reported that anticholinergic drugs antagonize the therapeutic effects of neuroleptics, but only with regard to positive symptoms.

Second, the exacerbation of schizophrenic (psychotic) symptoms induced by methylphenidate, a drug that increases dopaminergic activity, is reversed by physostigmine (Janowsky et al. 1973).

Third, physostigmine and other cholinergic agents may have transient and minor beneficial effects on psychotic symptoms (Pfeiffer and Jenney 1957; Rosenthal and Bigelow 1973).

Fourth, cholinergic agonists potentiate the effect of neuroleptics in the nucleus accumbens (Vance and Blumberg 1983). Increased dopaminergic activity in the nucleus accumbens and other limbic structures is postulated to be a major mechanism in the production of positive or "psychotic" schizophrenic symptoms.

Fifth, anticholinergic drugs have been reported to exacerbate "psychotic" symptoms in otherwise medication-free schizophrenic patients (Gershon and Olariu 1960; Itil et al. 1969). We recently studied the effects of biperiden (an anticholinergic agent) on 15 medication-free schizophrenic patients (Tandon et al. 1989d) and found that positive symptoms increased significantly ($t = 4.4$, 14 df, $P < .001$).

Finally, in most animal pharmaco-behavioral paradigms employed to assess antipsychotic activity, anticholinergic agents reverse actions of neuroleptics in a dose-dependent manner (Singh and Lal 1982).

COVARIANCE OF POSITIVE AND NEGATIVE SYMPTOMS IN PSYCHOTIC PHASE

Poor response to neuroleptics originally was considered to be one of the characteristic features of the negative schizophrenic syndrome (Crow 1980a; Andreasen 1982). There is no longer unanimity about this. The National Institute of Mental Health and Veterans Administration collaborative studies completed more than 20 years ago on the therapeutic effects of conventional neuroleptics (summarized in Cole et al. 1966) revealed considerable improvement in negative symptoms in a significant proportion of schizophrenic patients. The finding of improvement in negative symptoms during neuroleptic treatment also has been confirmed in recent studies (Breier et al. 1987; Goldberg 1985; Tandon et al. 1990b; van Kammen et al. 1987). Although negative symptoms respond to a lesser extent than do positive symptoms, the change in negative symptoms is significantly correlated to the change in positive symptoms. It also has been noted that there is an intensification of both positive and negative symptoms during a psychotic exacerbation in schizophrenia and a reduction in both as psychotic symptoms subside (Breier et al. 1987; Keefe et al. 1989). The concurrent increase of positive and negative symptoms during a psychotic exacerbation and their decline with neuroleptic treatment suggests that these phenomena may be caused by closely related processes, at least in this phase of the illness. Covariance of positive and negative symptoms is discussed elsewhere in this volume (Kay, Chapter 2; Pogue-Geile and Keshavan, Chapter 3).

HYPOTHESIZED MODEL OF CHOLINERGIC-DOPAMINERGIC INTERACTIONS

If positive symptoms are associated with decreasing cholinergic activity and negative symptoms with cholinergic hyperactivity, the covariance of positive and negative symptoms in the psychotic phase of schizophrenia is puzzling. In an effort to explain this paradox, we recently proposed a new model of dopaminergic-cholinergic interactions in schizophrenia (Tandon and Greden 1989). This model suggests that: 1) cholinergic-dopaminergic balance is of central importance in schizophrenic pathophysiology; 2) muscarinic activity increases in an attempt to maintain this balance in the face of increasing dopaminergic activity that occurs in the psychotic phase of the illness; 3) the muscarinic cholinergic system exerts a damping effect on the emergence of positive symptoms associated with dopaminergic hyperactivity; and 4) this compensatory increase in muscarinic activity is, in turn, accompanied by an intensification of negative symptoms during and following the psychotic phase of the illness.

The model is depicted in Figure 6-1 and is described in detail in Tandon and Greden (1989). The relationship of the model to different aspects and stages of schizophrenic psychopathology is now described.

Phenomenology of an Acute Psychotic Episode and Underlying Mechanisms

Limited data are available, but experts generally describe several distinct stages of schizophrenic decompensation and reintegration. Prior to the emergence of psychotic symptomatology, there appears to be a prepsychotic phase characterized by withdrawal, emotional blunting, boredom, lack of energy, depression, uneasiness, isolation, anhedonia, fatigue, and lassitude (Cameron 1938; Docherty et al. 1978; Donlon and Blacker 1973). "Depressive" symptoms commonly persist in the psychotic phase of the illness (Hirsch 1982; Knights et al. 1979), but are usually ignored because of the florid psychotic symptomatology. As psychotic symptoms remit, depressive symptoms are "revealed" or unmasked in what is commonly termed *postpsychotic depression* (Mandel et al. 1982; McGlashan and Carpenter 1976; Roth

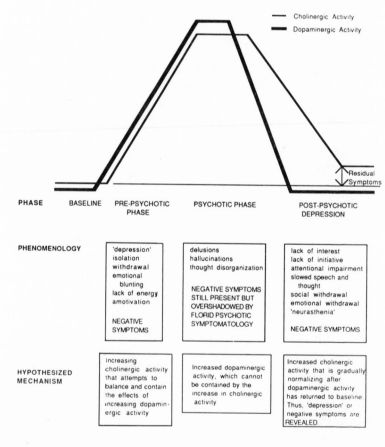

Figure 6-1. Cholinergic mechanisms and phenomenology of an acute psychotic episode.

1970) characterized by lack of interest, reduced initiative, attentional impairment, slowed speech and thought, social and emotional withdrawal, isolation, and "neurasthenic" symptomatology. The close resemblance of this profile to the negative schizophrenic syndrome is evident. The postpsychotic depressive phase lasts for several weeks before remitting gradually. Although the presence of depressive symptoms in the acute psychotic phase is generally considered to prognosticate a better outcome, their persistence long after the resolution of psychotic symptoms predicts a poor outcome (Mandel et al. 1982). Again, the similarity to the good prognostic import of negative symptoms in the acute phase and their bad prognostic import in the chronic stage of schizophrenia is striking.

These observations are consistent with the cholinergic hypothesis outlined below. The hypothesis proposes that mesolimbic cholinergic-dopaminergic balance is of central importance in schizophrenic pathophysiology, and that the cholinergic system exerts a damping or protective influence on the emergence of positive symptoms associated with dopaminergic hyperactivity. With the increase in dopaminergic activity at the outset of an acute psychotic episode, there occurs a compensatory increase in the activity of the cholinergic system in an effort to contain the effects of dopaminergic hyperactivity and prevent the expression of psychotic (positive) symptoms. This increase in cholinergic activity is accompanied by negative symptoms ("depressive" or withdrawal symptoms described in the process of decompensation to schizophrenic psychosis), a tendency to hypothalamic-pituitary-adrenal axis disinhibition (e.g., dexamethasone nonsuppression) and higher growth hormone response to thyrotropin-releasing hormone, and a likelihood of a better resolution of the present psychotic episode, since the increased cholinergic activity reflects an attempt to contain the psychopathologic effects of increased dopaminergic activity. The timing and implications of the neuroendocrine findings are discussed elsewhere (Keshavan et al., Chapter 8, this volume). Baseline sleep studies in this phase of the illness provide support for the existence of increased muscarinic activity. More recent sleep studies employing specific M-1 agonists (Berger et al. 1988, using RS-86) and antagonists (Tandon et al., in press a using biperiden) confirm muscarinic supersensitivity in this phase of the illness.

Cholinergic upregulation may be inadequate to prevent psychopathologic expression of increased dopaminergic activity in the form of positive symptoms, leading to the phase of acute psychotic symptomatology. There still would be a state of increased dopaminergic activity reflected in the persistent negative symptoms, which would be, however, obscured by the more prominent positive symptoms. Psychotic symptoms then might remit with or without neuroleptic treatment in association with a decrement in dopaminergic activity. Since cholinergic upregulation represents an attempt to contain effects of increased dopaminergic activity, anticholinergic agents would predictably exacerbate psychotic symptoms and antagonize the therapeutic efficacy of neuroleptic agents in this phase.

As dopaminergic activity declines in concordance with improvement in positive symptoms, the cholinergic system also begins to return to its "resting" or prepsychotic state; however, it normalizes at a slower rate because of its lesser plasticity, leading to prominent negative symptoms described as postpsychotic depression, revealed depression, or a phase of reintegration.

Cholinergic Mechanisms and Depressive Symptoms in Schizophrenia

Although depressive symptoms have been reported at various stages of schizophrenic illness, they are most commonly found before, during, and immediately after an acute psychotic exacerbation. The depressive symptoms most commonly reported are anergia, "neurasthenic" symptoms, slowed activity and thinking, and social and emotional withdrawal. It is apparent that this behavioral profile could as easily be labeled a negative symptom complex. These symptoms are in fact considered negative or residual "deficit" symptoms when they occur in the chronic phase of the illness. As previously described, the observed timing and course of depressive (negative ?) symptoms in schizophrenia are consistent with the postulated cholinergic hypothesis. Depressive symptoms in schizophrenia are occasionally responsive to imipramine and amitriptyline (Siris et al. 1978), antidepressants with considerable anticholinergic activity. Conversely, the clinical aphorism that antidepressants worsen schizophrenic (positive) symptomatology is also consistent with the proposed model.

Primary Versus Secondary Negative Symptoms

As discussed in Chapters 1–3, there may be difficulty in distinguishing "primary" negative symptoms from secondary negative symptoms due to extrapyramidal side effects of neuroleptics, to dysphoric affect or depression, to association with psychotic symptoms, or to understimulation. Two of these conditions (extrapyramidal side effects or parkinsonian symptoms, and depression) can also be caused by increased cholinergic activity (Dilsaver 1986; Duvoisin 1967), and negative symptoms associated with psychotic symptomatology may result from the compensatory cholinergic upregulation that occurs with positive symptoms and concomitant dopaminergic hyperactivity. Therefore, primary and secondary negative symptoms could have the same pathophysiologic basis (i.e., cholinergic hyperactivity), making it difficult to distinguish between them. Treatment response can also be misleading: "parkinsonian" negative symptoms (akinetic depression) would respond to anticholinergic agents, "depressive" negative symptoms may respond to treatment with antidepressants because of their anticholinergic activity (Kasper et al. 1981), and "primary" negative symptoms have been seen to respond to anticholinergic treatment in the absence of parkinsonian or depressive symptoms (Fayen et al. 1988; Tandon et al. 1988). This issue obviously needs further exploration.

Cholinergic Mechanisms and the Heterogeneity of Schizophrenia

Several schemes have been proposed to seek order within the heterogeneity maze of schizophrenia. The most prominent of these are the positive-negative syndrome dichotomy and the paranoid-nonparanoid dichotomy. The cholinergic hypothesis may contribute to an explanation of these dichotomies.

Positive-Negative Dichotomy. Positive and negative syndromes may have distinct but related underlying mechanisms (dopaminergic and cholinergic hyperactivity, respectively), thereby accounting for their distinct but related biological associations, treatment response, and longitudinal course.

Paranoid-Nonparanoid Dichotomy. Nonparanoid schizophrenic patients have been found to be sensitive to anticholinergic reversal of the therapeutic effects of neuroleptics, but paranoid schizophrenic patients reportedly are not (Singh et al. 1987). Our hypothesis would suggest that while the cholinergic system upregulates in nonparanoid patients (leading to anticholinergic exacerbation of positive symptoms), it may not do so in paranoid patients. The failure of cholinergic upregulation in paranoid patients may explain their worse "positive-symptom" outcome (persistence of paranoid symptomatology because of no increase in cholinergic activity to contain the effects of dopaminergic hyperactivity), but better social outcome due to less prominent negative symptoms (no increase in cholinergic activity).

Neurobiologic Basis of Proposed Dopaminergic-Cholinergic Interactions

The parts of the brain commonly linked to schizophrenia (the hippocampus, nucleus accumbens, amygdala, septal nuclei, other parts of the limbic system, and the dorsolateral prefrontal cortex) are richly supplied by septal-hippocampal, cortical, and other cholinergic pathways (Robinson 1985). There is considerable evidence for significant reciprocal interactions between the dopamine and acetylcholine pathways in these regions. Although the precise nature of these interactions is unclear, cholinergic-dopaminergic balance is described as being of critical homeostatic importance. An increase in dopaminergic activity (from a variety of causes) results in a compensatory increase in muscarinic activity (Beani and Bianchi 1973; Costall and Naylor 1972; Pepeu and Bartolini 1968). This "cholinergic counteraction" is mediated specifically by D_2 dopamine receptors (Casamenti et al. 1987), a fact of considerable interest in view of the dopamine D_2 receptor increase reported in schizophrenia (Owen et al. 1978) and the association between the antipsychotic potency of neuroleptics and their D_2 blocking activity (Creese et al. 1976; Richelson 1984; Seeman et al. 1976). Although the nature of dopamine-acetylcholine interactions in the brain areas of interest needs to be further clarified, these networks and interactions may provide the neurobiologic substrate of the model described.

SUMMARY AND CRITIQUE

We have presented phenomenological, pharmacologic, behavioral, neuroendocrine, polysomnographic, and other evidence suggesting that muscarinic hyperactivity may be an important mechanism in the production of negative schizophrenic symptoms, particularly in the acute psychotic phase of the illness. This mechanism may be involved in the pathogenesis of primary negative symptoms, as well as of negative symptoms "secondary" to depression, parkinsonian side effects of neuroleptics, and psychotic symptomatology. We also have reviewed data suggesting a worsening of positive symptoms when cholinergic activity is decreased in the acute psychotic phase of schizophrenia. On the basis of this evidence, we have hypothesized that cholinergic-dopaminergic balance is of central importance in schizophrenic pathophysiology and that the cholinergic system may exert a damping effect on the emergence of positive symptoms associated with dopaminergic hyperactivity. This increase in limbic cholinergic activity is accompanied by negative or "depressive" symptoms before, during, and immediately after a psychotic episode. Failure of the cholinergic system to return to baseline may be an important mechanism in the production of residual negative or "deficit" symptoms. Fluctuations in cholinergic activity at different stages of schizophrenia may partially explain the longitudinal course and prognosis of schizophrenic illness and may, in part, help to explain the variability and heterogeneity of schizophrenia.

Furthermore, dorsolateral prefrontal cortical dysfunction, cerebral atrophy, and other structural brain changes have been implicated in the production of negative symptoms. Perinatal injury and infection have also been suggested as important etiologic mechanisms. (It should be noted that the implicated brain areas are richly innervated by cholinergic fibers and that the cholinergic system is extremely sensitive to anoxic and other injury.) These mechanisms are probably interrelated, with some more immediately involved in schizophrenic pathophysiology and others more peripheral, representing epiphenomena.

We emphasize that we are not proposing an exclusive mono-transmitter (cholinergic) hypothesis of negative symptoms or schizophrenia. Such approaches are outdated. Indeed, dopaminergic mechanisms are obviously important, serotonergic and noradrenergic mechanisms have been linked with negative symptoms, and other neurotransmitters may be involved as well. Exactly how these systems may interact remains unclear. Cholinergic hyperactivity may be involved in the production of negative symptoms in a subgroup of schizophrenic patients; alternatively, cholinergic interactions with other neurotransmitter systems may be important in the pathogenesis of negative schizophrenic symptoms in certain phases of the illness.

The hypothesis suggested is supported indirectly by data from several lines of research, is internally consistent, is congruent with current knowledge about schizophrenia, and may explain some apparently discrepant findings. Despite the sketchiness of current evidence, it probably is reasonable to pursue further the hypothesis that the cholinergic system plays a role in schizophrenic pathophysiology and that muscarinic hyperactivity may be an important mechanism in the production of negative schizophrenic symptoms.

Chapter 7

Noradrenergic Mechanisms, State Dependency, and Negative Symptoms in Schizophrenia

Daniel P. van Kammen, M.D., Ph.D.
Jeffrey L. Peters, M.D.
Jeffrey Yao, Ph.D.
Welmoet B. van Kammen, Ph.D.
Thomas Neylan, M.D.
David Shaw, Ph.D.

Chapter 7

Noradrenergic Mechanisms, State Dependency, and Negative Symptoms in Schizophrenia

Most investigators now acknowledge the limitations of the dopamine hypothesis of schizophrenia and its inability to explain all psychopathology (Carlsson 1988). At the same time, there is increasing evidence to support a role for norepinephrine in schizophrenic psychopathology (Hornykiewicz 1982; van Kammen et al. 1987). Hypotheses implicating norepinephrine in negative symptoms emerged almost two decades ago. Stein and Wise (1971) proposed that anhedonia and loss of drive were due to the deterioration of central noradrenergic reward pathways, as indicated by decreased dopamine-beta-hydroxylase levels (DBH). In addition, elevated norepinephrine levels have been consistently reported to be present in the cerebral spinal fluid (CSF) of drug-free schizophrenic patients (Beckmann et al. 1983; Gomes et al. 1980; Kemali et al. 1982; Lake et al. 1980; Sternberg et al. 1981) and in brains at autopsy (Bird et al. 1979; Bridge et al. 1985; Crow et al. 1979; Farley et al.

We gratefully acknowledge the support and collaborations of Ms. Doris McAdam, R.N., head nurse, her nursing staff, and the patients of the Schizophrenia Research Unit at the Highland Drive VAMC, Pittsburgh, PA. Parts of this manuscript were presented at the Negative Symptom Symposium at the American Psychiatric Association Meeting, Montreal, Canada, May 1988 and at the Negative Symptom Symposium at the Regional Meeting of the World Psychiatric Association in Washington, DC, October 1988. The assistance of Mary Kelley, B.S., in preparation of this manuscript is gratefully acknowledged. Partial funding for this research was provided by the Highland Drive VAMC and the Veterans Administration Research Service to Dr. van Kammen.

1978, 1979). In fact, elevated norepinephrine levels are among the most consistently replicated findings in the biochemical studies of schizophrenic patients (Hornykiewicz 1982; van Kammen and Gelernter 1987). Whereas decreased CSF DBH appears to be quite stable over time (Sternberg et al. 1982, 1983), CSF norepinephrine appears to vary state-dependently in schizophrenic patients (Linnoila et al. 1983; van Kammen et al. 1985b), being higher during a psychotic exacerbation.

Studying negative symptoms is difficult; a key reason is the lack of agreement as to what constitutes a negative symptom (as discussed in detail in chapters in the first section of this volume). Most investigators agree, however, about one aspect of negative symptoms: their irreversibility. According to Crow (1980a), the negative symptom syndrome (Type II), once it develops, is a stable characteristic of schizophrenia; he included such features as lateral ventricle enlargement, poor premorbid functioning, and neuroleptic nonresponsiveness in the Type II syndrome. While several groups have been able to show an association between wide ventricles and negative symptoms (Andreasen and Olsen 1982; Smith et al. 1984; van Kammen et al. 1988), suggesting a neuroanatomical basis for stable negative symptoms or the deficit syndrome in schizophrenia (Levin 1984; van Kammen et al. 1988; Weinberger 1987), other groups have been unable to link negative symptoms with brain atrophy (Bishop et al. 1983; Luchins et al. 1984; Nasrallah et al. 1983b; van Kammen et al. 1983, 1986b).

By contrast, Johnstone et al. (1987) showed in a longitudinal study that negative symptoms in chronic patients are less stable than positive symptoms, supporting the proposition that negative symptoms do in fact change. Goldberg et al. (1967) had shown that negative symptoms can decrease with neuroleptics. Since then, reports that negative symptoms respond to neuroleptic treatment have appeared (Rosen et al. 1984; van Kammen et al. 1987). The confusion about whether negative symptoms in schizophrenia are drug responsive may result from differences in the clinical phase of study. One way to resolve these inconsistencies is to categorize negative symptoms as drug responsive, drug nonresponsive (or residual), and drug-induced (van Kammen et al. 1987). Unfortunately, as discussed in the first section of this volume, it is difficult to separate these symptoms phenomenologically, particularly because there are so many definitions of negative symptoms (Carpenter et al. 1988; Liddle 1987a). Conceivably, some confusion may derive from treating negative symptoms as a categorical rather than as a dimensional variable (i.e., Type II versus Type I schizophrenia) (Meltzer 1984).

Studies of the relapse process have indicated that negative symptoms can emerge as prodromal symptoms or may remain as residual symptoms (Docherty et al. 1978; Herz and Melville 1980) (Table 7-1). When acutely psychotic patients require treatment, negative symptoms are of less concern than the agitation, hallucinations, delusions, or anxiety, which the clinician expects to treat successfully with antipsychotic drugs. After the patients have been optimally treated for their positive symptoms, however, residual negative symptoms become the major concern. Actually, a decrease in apparently drug-induced psychotic symptoms is sometimes observed in clinically stable patients after withdrawal of antipsychotic agents (Marder et al. 1979; Naber et al. 1985; van Kammen et al.

Table 7-1. Stages of schizophrenic decompensation and reintegration: Negative and prodromal symptoms

	Norepinephrine
I. *Overextension — stressed* Distractibility Attentional deficits	↑
II. *Restricted consciousness* Flat affect, anhedonia Apathy, listlessness Attentional deficit Social withdrawal	↑ or ↓
III. *Prepsychotic state — disinhibition* Hypomania Loss of sleep Hyperactivity, hypervigilance Increased anxiety Increased sexual feelings Increased psychotic symptoms	↑
IV. *Psychotic disorganization* Positive symptoms Disintegration of higher functioning Flat affect Emotional and social withdrawal	↑
V. *Psychotic resolution* Poor self-care Decreased anxiety	= or ↓

Source. Adapted from Docherty et al. (1978).

1990). Even though these patients may need antipsychotic medication again later to control positive symptoms after relapse (Marder et al. 1979; van Putten et al. 1974), they may benefit from lower than traditional doses of medication (Marder et al. 1979).

If one accepts that negative symptom severity in a patient who is not in a chronic deficit state (Type II) may be state dependent, then it becomes understandable that the clinical status of the patients in a given study sample will determine whether relationships between negative symptoms and brain atrophy or medication-responsiveness will be observed. For example, the relationship between negative symptoms and computed tomography scan abnormalities will most likely be seen in a group of clinically stable, chronic schizophrenic patients with poor response to neuroleptic drugs.

We have reported previously that CSF norepinephrine levels can be state dependent in schizophrenic patients (van Kammen et al. 1981, 1985b, 1989, 1990). We also observed that negative symptoms were increased in relapsed patients who subsequently responded to pimozide (van Kammen et al. 1987), while pimozide treatment decreased CSF norepinephrine in parallel with the decrease in psychotic symptoms (Sternberg et al. 1981). These observations, taken together, suggest that the increase in negative symptoms noted in relapsed patients is associated with increases in CSF norepinephrine and 3-methoxy-4-hydroxyphenylglycol (MHPG) levels.

NORADRENERGIC MECHANISMS

To examine the role of norepinephrine in negative symptoms, we evaluated CSF monoamines and negative symptom ratings in a group of stable, chronic schizophrenic patients before and after they were withdrawn from haloperidol maintenance treatment. We hypothesized that increased CSF norepinephrine would be associated with increased negative symptoms in relapsed patients, based on the observation that relapsed patients have both increased negative symptoms (van Kammen et al. 1987) and elevated CSF norepinephrine levels (van Kammen et al. 1989). In clinically stable patients, we expected to observe negative relationships between negative symptoms and CSF norepinephrine. We propose that clinical heterogeneity in schizophrenia may be caused by different expressions of a norepinephrine dysregulation over time. The study design is described in detail elsewhere (van Kammen et al. 1990).

We studied 32 DSM-III-R (American Psychiatric Association 1987) schizophrenic inpatients on neuroleptic treatment at the Schizophrenia Research Unit of the Highland Drive Veterans Administration Medical Center in Pittsburgh, Pennsylvania. Their mean

(±SD) age was 34.2 ± 7.6 years. Eighteen patients were diagnosed as having paranoid schizophrenia, 10 as having undifferentiated schizophrenia, and 4 as having schizoaffective disorder, mainly schizophrenic. Premorbid functioning was assessed with the Premorbid Adjustment Scale (Cannon-Spoor et al. 1982). Neuroleptic dosage was converted to haloperidol equivalents in all patients who were not already being treated with haloperidol. Following stabilization on the lowest therapeutic dose of haloperidol, patients entered a double-blind medication phase. After several weeks of treatment with haloperidol, patients received placebo for up to 6 weeks. All patients were maintained on a low-monamine, caffeine-restricted, and alcohol-free diet during hospitalization. Patients did not receive sedatives, antianxiety drugs, or any other medication during the time they were in the study. A lumbar puncture was performed on all patients during the last week on haloperidol treatment. In the drug-free condition, a lumbar puncture was performed on relapsers within days of meeting relapse criteria (see below) (22 ± 3 days drug-free) and on nonrelapsers at the end of the 6 weeks on placebo. Standard procedures for collection and storage of CSF were followed and assays for norepinephrine, MHPG, homovanillac acid (HVA), and 5-hydroxyindoleacetic acid (5-HIAA) were conducted using the high performance liquid chromatography method described by Scheinin et al. (1983). Patients were rated weekly with the Scale for the Assessment of Negative Symptoms (SANS) (Andreasen 1982), the Brief Psychiatric Rating Scale (BPRS) (Overall et al. 1963), and the 15-point global psychosis rating scale (Bunney and Hamburg 1963). A mean increase of 3 points on the global psychosis ratings over 3 days (van Kammen et al. 1982) and an increase of 10 points in the BPRS psychosis subscale (Lieberman et al. 1987) were taken to indicate relapse. After haloperidol withdrawal, 14 patients relapsed within 6 weeks; 18 did not. Statistical analyses included comparisons of haloperidol versus drug-free conditions and of relapsers versus nonrelapsers, using Student's *t* tests (two-tailed significance) and Pearson correlation coefficients (two-tailed significance).

Our findings are summarized in Table 7-2, which shows the relationships between negative symptoms as measured by the SANS and CSF measures in drug-free schizophrenic patients (i.e., withdrawn from haloperidol). CSF norepinephrine and MHPG correlated significantly with negative symptom subscales, but CSF HVA and 5-HIAA did not.

Differences Between Relapsers and Nonrelapsers

There were no significant differences between relapsers and nonrelapsers in age, age at onset of illness, duration of illness, premorbid adjustment, or daily haloperidol dose. Relapsers and nonrelapsers did not differ significantly in their negative symptom ratings during haloperidol treatment. In the drug-free phase, however, all negative symptom subscales as well as the total scores were significantly higher in the relapsers (Table 7-3). Relapsers had significantly higher CSF norepinephrine levels before and after haloperidol withdrawal. CSF MHPG was significantly higher in relapsers only after haloperidol withdrawal. CSF HVA and 5-HIAA concentrations did not differ between the two groups at either time point (Table 7-4). When correlations between CSF variables and negative symptoms were computed on relapsers and nonrelapsers separately, relapsers showed a significant positive correlation between CSF norepinephrine and

Table 7-2. Drug-free CSF and negative symptoms for all patients: Correlations between CSF amine metabolites and negative symptom subscales

	NE	MHPG	HVA	5-HIAA	PSYCH
Affective flattening					
r	.46	.45	.026	.17	.54
P	.012	.013	NS	NS	0.001
Alogia					
r	.46	.35	−.053	.13	.67
P	.011	.059	NS	NS	.000
Avolition-apathy					
r	.34	.21	.10	.17	.49
P	.073	NS	NS	NS	.004
Anhedonia-asociality					
r	.53	.46	.05	.23	.79
P	.003	.011	NS	NS	.000
Attentional deficit					
r	.47	.41	.02	.28	.58
P	.009	.026	NS	NS	.000
Total score					
r	.50	.41	.03	.22	.69
P	.006	.024	NS	NS	.000
Psychosis					
r	.56	.50	−.10	.07	*
P	.001	.005	NS	NS	

Note. Correlations are two-tailed. CSF = cerebrospinal fluid. NE = norepinephrine. MHPG = 3-methoxy-4-hydroxyphenylglycol. HVA = homovanillic acid. 5-HIAA = 5-hydroxyindoleacetic acid. PSYCH = psychosis rating the day before the lumbar puncture, Bunney and Hamburg (1963) scale. NS = $P > .10$.

MHPG on the one hand and measures of negative symptoms, psychosis, and global ratings on the other (Table 7-5). Nonrelapsers showed no significant correlations, although there was a nonsignificant negative relationship between CSF norepinephrine and MHPG on the one hand and negative symptom ratings on the other (r = -.08 to -.41, NS).

Changes Between Haloperidol and Drug-Free Phases

Negative symptoms increased significantly in the relapsed patients following haloperidol withdrawal but showed no significant change in the stable patients. Changes in CSF norepinephrine and MHPG did not correlate significantly with changes in negative symptom scores following haloperidol withdrawal, except for changes in CSF

Table 7-3. Severity of negative symptoms in relapsers and nonrelapsers in drug-free phase

	Relapsers	Nonrelapsers	t	P
Affective flattening	2.3 ± 1.21	1.2 ± 0.80	2.92	.008
Alogia	2.3 ± 1.33	0.7 ± 1.01	3.82	.001
Avolition-apathy	2.3 ± 1.15	1.2 ± 0.95	2.90	.007
Anhedonia-asociality	3.3 ± 0.84	1.7 ± 0.82	5.51	.0001
Attentional impairment	2.3 ± 1.39	1.1 ± 1.18	2.74	.010
Total score	12.7 ± 5.36	6.0 ± 3.79	4.09	.0001
Psychosis	10.4 ± 1.65	4.1 ± 1.78	10.28	.0001

Table 7-4. Cerebrospinal fluid levels: Drug condition and relapse

	Relapsers	Nonrelapsers	t	P
Haloperidol phase				
NE	.79 ± .36	.52 ± .35	2.15	.04
MHPG	35.1 ± 7.17	34.3 ± 7.65	.31	NS
HVA	164.5 ± 62.3	175.6 ± 66.6	−.45	NS
5-HIAA	100.9 ± 43.7	82.1 ± 25.2	1.39	NS
Drug-free phase				
NE	.91 ± .51	.48 ± .28	2.73	.01
MHPG	46.2 ± 16.8	35.4 ± 8.89	2.04	.05
HVA	162.4 ± 87.5	202.5 ± 142.8	−.87	NS
5-HIAA	103.6 ± 31.4	99.5 ± 47.0	.26	NS

Note. NE = norepinephrine. MHPG = 3-methoxy-4-hydroxyphenylglycol. HVA = homovanillic acid. 5-HIAA = 5-hydroxyindoleacetic acid.

MHPG and anhedonia (N = 29, r = .45, P = .01). Changes in CSF
MHPG showed a trend toward a significant correlation with changes
in total SANS (r = .32, P = .09) and inattentiveness (r = .33, P = .07)
scores; likewise, changes in CSF norepinephrine showed a trend
toward a significant correlation with changes in total SANS scores
(r = .35, P = .06), alogia (r = .33, P = .08), inattentiveness (r = .33,
P = .08), and anhedonia (r = .33, P = .08).

DISCUSSION

Although several methodological issues merit attention, our data
indicate the following. First, at the time of the drug-free lumbar
puncture, CSF norepinephrine and MHPG increased, whereas CSF
HVA did not. Second, negative symptom ratings correlated positively
and significantly with CSF norepinephrine and MHPG but not with
CSF HVA or 5-HIAA. These correlations were significant only in

Table 7-5. Relationship between CSF amine metabolites and
negative symptoms in relapsers in the drug-free phase

	NE	MHPG	HVA	5-HIAA	PSYCH
Affective flattening					
r	.41	.37	−.20	−.06	.42
P	NS	NS	NS	NS	NS
Alogia					
r	.50	.43	−.079	−.11	.66
P	.076	NS	NS	NS	.011
Avolition-apathy					
r	.40	.28	.06	−.04	.24
P	NS	NS	NS	NS	NS
Anhedonia-asociality					
r	.52	.70	.33	.36	.55
P	.068	.012	NS	NS	.044
Attentional deficit					
r	.60	.62	.10	.12	.66
P	.031	.030	NS	NS	.010
Total score					
r	.54	.52	.03	.04	.57
P	.059	.085	NS	NS	.035
Psychosis					
r	.57	.73	.34	.35	*
P	.040	.008	NS	NS	

Note. Correlations are two-tailed. CSF = cerebrospinal fluid. NE = norepinephrine.
MHPG = 3-methoxy-4-hydroxyphenylglycol. HVA = homovanillic acid. 5-HIAA
= 5-hydroxyindoleacetic acid. PSYCH = psychosis rating before the lumbar puncture, Bunney and Hamburg (1963) scale. NS = P > .10.

patients who relapsed after discontinuation of haloperidol. Third, relapse following haloperidol withdrawal was associated with increases in negative symptoms and CSF norepinephrine and MHPG concentrations, but only in those who relapsed following haloperidol withdrawal. Fourth, consistent with the Stein and Wise (1971) hypothesis, after haloperidol withdrawal, negative symptoms and CSF norepinephrine or MHPG correlated negatively in the nonrelapsers, albeit nonsignificantly. This finding suggests that the deficit syndrome or residual symptoms may be associated with decreased norepinephrine activity, particularly those symptoms that might result from loss of behaviors maintained by operant conditioning, in which norepinephrine activity plays a role (Morley et al. 1988). Finally, increased noradrenergic activity may be associated with increases in negative and positive symptoms in the psychotic phase, whereas residual negative symptoms are associated with decreased central nervous system noradrenergic activity.

CSF norepinephrine appears to be less stable than CSF MHPG, HVA, or 5-HIAA when sampled in the same patients over several drug-free evaluations (Linnoila et al. 1983); it has also been shown (above) to be correlated with severity of psychosis. These observations support the suggestion that CSF norepinephrine levels are state-dependent (van Kammen et al. 1985b). Because sleep can decrease as a behavioral prodrome to psychotic decompensation (Docherty et al. 1978; Herz and Melville 1980) (Figure 7-1), the relationship of duration of sleep the night before the lumbar puncture with CSF norepinephrine was tested and found to be negative and highly significant ($N = 53$, $r = -.44$, $P < .0008$) (van Kammen and Antelman 1984), lending further support to the hypothesis that CSF norepinephrine levels may lead to state-dependent changes in behavior (van Kammen et al. 1985b).

Differentiation of Negative Symptoms

A positive relationship between positive and negative symptoms has been observed by some investigators (Bishop et al. 1983; Nasrallah et al. 1983b; Rosen et al. 1984; van Kammen et al. 1987), although not by others (Andreasen 1985; Stahl et al. 1985). This finding may result from differences in sample characteristics or other methodological factors described in Chapters 2 and 4 of this volume. Relapsed patients, in whom negative symptoms have been shown to increase (Rosen et al. 1984; van Kammen et al. 1987), may be less likely to participate in studies. Therefore, conclusions about the effects of neuroleptic withdrawal are often drawn from results in a sample of largely stable patients, in whom the relationship may be masked. We suggest that as long as the nature and etiology of negative symptoms remains unclear, categorizing negative symptoms as drug responsive, drug nonresponsive, or drug-induced, as has been done for positive symptoms (Marder et al. 1979; van Putten et al. 1974), may help to explain the conflicting data (van Kammen et al. 1987, 1988).

Can Increased Norepinephrine and Negative Symptoms Be Prodromes of Relapse?

We have shown previously that biochemical as well as behavioral prodromes of relapse could be identified in schizophrenia (van Kammen et al. 1982). The behavioral prodrome is similar to the profile of the negative syndrome and is accompanied by an increase in norepinephrine (Table 7-1). In the study described above, we found that CSF MHPG was increased significantly in drug-free relapsers and correlated significantly with psychosis ratings ($N = 28$, $r = .49$, $P < .004$) and sleep ($N = 27$, $r = .55$, $P < .001$) (van Kammen et al. 1986a). CSF HVA or 5-HIAA levels, however, did not differ significantly between relapsers and nonrelapsers, nor did these values change with haloperidol withdrawal. We also found that CSF norepinephrine was elevated in relapsers in both the drug-free state (Figure 7-2) and prior to haloperidol withdrawal (Figure 7-3). Similarly, negative symptoms and psychosis ratings increased significantly between the haloperidol

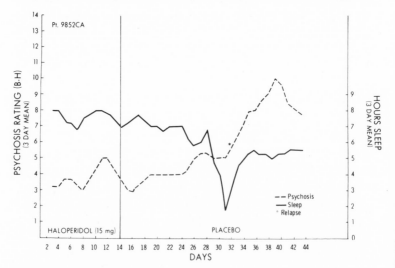

Figure 7-1. Relationship between sleep and psychotic exacerbation. B-H = Bunney and Hamburg (1963) scale.

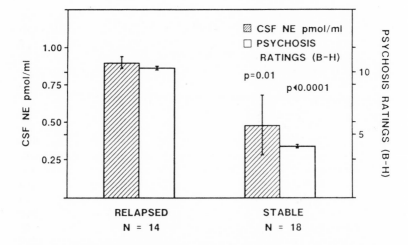

Figure 7-2. Cerebrospinal fluid (CSF) norepinephrine (NE) and psychosis in drug-free schizophrenic patients. B-H = Bunney and Hamburg (1963) scale.

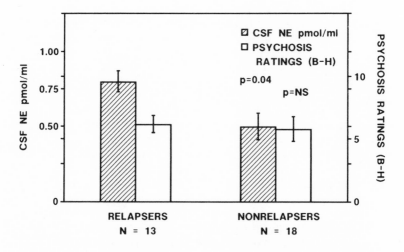

Figure 7-3. Cerebrospinal fluid (CSF) norepinephrine (NE) and psychosis in haloperidol-treated schizophrenic patients. B-H = Bunney and Hamburg (1963) scale.

and the drug-free states in the relapsers (Table 7-3), but not in the nonrelapsers. When we compared relapsers with nonrelapsers prior to haloperidol withdrawal, no significant differences in CSF measures, psychosis ratings, or duration of sleep were found. CSF norepinephrine and MHPG correlated significantly with psychosis ratings and sleep the night before the lumbar puncture in the drug-free state (Table 7-2), supporting our hypothesis that the increase in norepinephrine occurred prior to rather than subsequent to the increase in psychosis. In a recent study, Pickar et al. (1990) observed that CSF MHPG levels were significantly elevated in 22 drug-free schizophrenic inpatients and that negative symptoms were best correlated with plasma MHPG, further suggesting noradrenergic relationships to negative symptoms and psychotic processes. Taken together, these findings suggest that an increase in negative symptoms, disturbed sleep, and increase in norepinephrine may be a prodrome of a psychotic relapse.

Noradrenergic Modulation of Symptoms

The positive relationships of CSF norepinephrine and CSF MHPG with negative symptom ratings suggest that negative symptoms may be aggravated by increased norepinephrine activity. Since we observed similar significant relationships with positive symptoms and covariance of positive and negative symptoms in this group, we propose that increased norepinephrine activity may turn up the "gain"—that is, increase the base rate of symptoms regardless of whether they are positive or negative. Presumably CSF norepinephrine and MHPG originate from the locus coeruleus, and our data are, in fact, consistent with one of the roles of the locus coeruleus, regulating the output of target neurons (Foote et al. 1983). Our data suggest that the norepinephrine disturbance may not have a primary etiologic significance in relapsed schizophrenic patients, but rather may amplify symptom change (van Kammen and Antelman 1984; van Kammen et al. 1981), presumably by bringing out the underlying dopamine disturbance. Increasing "gain" is a well-documented function of norepinephrine in the central nervous system (Antelman and Caggiula 1977; Foote et al. 1983) and is consistent with the possibility that shifts in norepinephrine activity regulate or modify the intensity of symptoms produced by a primary disturbance. In all likelihood, this primary disturbance in schizophrenia involves faulty dopamine regulation (Carlsson 1988), although other systems such as serotonin (Friedhoff 1988; Stahl et al. 1985) have also been implicated.

Primary Role for Noradrenergic Dysregulation in Schizophrenic Symptomatology

In clinically stable patients, however, negative symptoms were found to correlate negatively with CSF norepinephrine and MHPG at both phases, suggesting a more direct etiologic role for norepinephrine in negative symptomatology in these patients. Presumably, decreased norepinephrine activity may be associated with the defect state in schizophrenia, in accordance with the hypotheses of neuronal loss (Stein and Wise 1971). There is additional evidence suggesting that norepinephrine activity may indeed have a primary role in schizophrenia. Lohr and Jeste (1988) reported that the cell volume of the locus coeruleus of DSM-III (American Psychiatric Association 1980) schizophrenic patients was significantly decreased. This finding, which requires replication, is consistent with the reported decrease in CSF DBH in patients with evidence of brain atrophy (van Kammen et al. 1983), but seemingly inconsistent with the reported increase in CSF norepinephrine in relapsed patients (Figure 7-3). Norepinephrine, however, can be released by noradrenergic neurons independently from DBH release, which is quite stable (Sternberg et al. 1982), whereas norepinephrine levels fluctuate with clinical state independently from DBH (Linnoila et al. 1983). Furthermore, as discussed above, this increase in norepinephrine is probably a state-dependent phenomenon.

A review of the literature suggests that brain atrophy in schizophrenia may reflect a brain lesion, the cause of which may have to be sought prior to the onset of illness (Goetz and van Kammen 1986), if it is not secondary to perinatal trauma or anoxia (Foerster et al., Chapter 12, this volume; Murray et al. 1986). Conceivably, patients with brain atrophy could have a poorly regulated norepinephrine system that responds to stress either too strongly or not at all. We have reported a negative relationship in our National Institute of Mental Health patient sample between CSF norepinephrine and cortical atrophy ($r = -.29$, $P < .04$) and not with ventricle-to-brain ratio ($r = -.04$, $P = $ NS) (van Kammen et al. 1985a), which provides further evidence that decreased noradrenergic activity may be present in the deficit syndrome.

Negative Symptoms and Neuroleptic Treatment Response

We propose that negative and positive symptoms respond to neuroleptic treatment (Goldberg 1985; van Kammen et al. 1987) only in the presence of elevated noradrenergic activity (e.g., CSF norepinephrine [Sternberg et al. 1981], CSF MHPG [Sedvall et al.

1976], or plasma MHPG [Bowers et al. 1987]). Results of several investigations support this hypothesis. Sternberg et al. (1981) reported that the decrease in CSF norepinephrine associated with pimozide treatment paralleled a decrease in psychosis. This decrease in CSF norepinephrine is consistent with the findings of Dinan and Aston-Jones (1985), who noted that chronic haloperidol treatment decreased the firing rate of noradrenergic neurons in the locus coeruleus. This decrease is not, however, a depolarization inactivation as observed in the dopamine system (Grace and Bunney 1980). In another study of pimozide treatment in relapsed schizophrenic patients, van Kammen et al. (1987) found that pretreatment negative symptoms were higher in the pimozide responders than in the non-responders. Negative symptoms decreased as much as positive symptoms. A more detailed review of the relationships between pretreatment catecholaminergic activity and treatment response can be found elsewhere (van Kammen et al. 1989).

Norepinephrine and Dopamine Interactions

Several groups have shown that dopamine and norepinephrine cells communicate with each other, either directly or through intermediary cells (Anisman et al. 1981; Antelman and Caggiula 1977; Bunney and DeRiemer 1982; Glowinski et al. 1988; Grenhoff and Svennson 1988; Ornstein et al. 1987). Actually, a functionally active norepinephrine system is needed to express D_1 receptor supersensitivity following lesions in the dopamine system (Glowinski et al. 1988), while norepinephrine activity affects apomorphine-induced stereotypes (Dickinson et al. 1988).

CSF norepinephrine and dopamine have been found to correlate significantly in drug-free schizophrenic patients (Gattaz et al. 1983; Kemali et al. 1982; van Kammen and Antelman 1984). Moreover, indirect dopaminergic agents that aggravate schizophrenic symptoms (e.g., d-amphetamine, methylphenidate, and L-dopa) also increase norepinephrine release (van Kammen and Antelman 1984). These findings indicate that norepinephrine may influence schizophrenia in conjunction with a dopamine disturbance. Although acute receptor blockade increases dopamine and norepinephrine levels, chronic neuroleptic treatment decreases the firing rate of dopamine (Grace and Bunney 1980) and norepinephrine (Dinan and Aston-Jones 1985) cells, which could explain the reported decreases in CSF HVA (Bowers and Rozitis 1974; Post et al. 1975), plasma HVA (Chang et al. 1988; Davila et al. 1988), and CSF norepinephrine (Sternberg et al. 1981) that are observed with chronic antipsychotic drug treatment. Furthermore, neuroleptics block the inhibitory effects of norepinephrine on cerebellar Purkinje cells relative to their antipsychotic efficacy (Freedman 1977), which parallels the observed relationship between D_2 receptor blockade and clinical potency (Creese et al. 1976; Seeman and Lee 1975).

CONCLUSIONS

Although dopamine activity is integrally involved in schizophrenic symptomatology, disturbances in norepinephrine activity are present as well. Our findings suggest that increased norepinephrine release in schizophrenic patients may amplify positive and negative symptoms during a relapse. Furthermore, increased norepinephrine activity may trigger a disturbance in dopamine activity that leads to increased psychosis and negative symptoms. The contention of Hornykiewicz (1982) that increased norepinephrine activity plays an important role in schizophrenia appears to be valid.

Our data do not provide an explanation for neuroleptic nonresponsive symptoms or the deficit syndrome, even though there is a hint in the form of a possible relationship between decreased norepinephrine and negative symptoms in stable patients, suggesting that norepinephrine activity may be decreased in the residual or deficit syndrome. In this regard, decreases in norepinephrine (or dopamine) activity may be insufficient to render most patients asymptomatic, and negative symptoms may actually worsen because of this decrease. Whether this possibility accounts for the relationships among negative symptoms, poor drug response, and brain atrophy remains to be explored.

Chapter 8

Positive and Negative Symptoms and Neuroendocrine Dysfunction in Schizophrenia

Matcheri S. Keshavan, M.D.
Cheryl Mazzara, M.D.
J. Brar, M.D.
John F. Dequardo, M.D.

Chapter 8

Positive and Negative Symptoms and Neuroendocrine Dysfunction in Schizophrenia

Endocrine factors have long been considered relevant to schizophrenia. Reasons for this assumption have included the onset of schizophrenia in adolescence and the association between schizophrenic symptoms and puerperium, menopause, and the premenstrual period. As will be indicated in this review, a variety of neuroendocrine alterations have been described in schizophrenia. To place findings in proper perspective, it should be noted that endocrine factors are unlikely to be primary in the etiology of schizophrenia, because 1) no evidence exists of a specific endocrine disorder occurring regularly in schizophrenic patients, and 2) schizophrenia-like psychopathology is the exception rather than the rule in endocrine disease (Bleuler 1964). It is more likely that endocrine changes reflect altered brain neurotransmitter function in some schizophrenic patients, the likely reason being the clinical and biological heterogeneity of the schizophrenic syndrome.

As reflected throughout this volume, patients with "positive and negative" syndromes may differ in neurochemical pathology. If so, one could hypothesize neuroendocrine differences between schizophrenic patients based on this dichotomy. We will review the neuroendocrinology of schizophrenia with regard to this question. More exhaustive reviews of other aspects of psychoneuroendocrine changes in patients with schizophrenia can be found elsewhere (Ferrier 1987; Powchik et al. 1987).

ANTERIOR PITUITARY HORMONES

Prolactin

Prolactin secretion is tonically inhibited by dopamine. Since dopamine in the central nervous system has been implicated in the pathophysiology of schizophrenia, measurement of prolactin has gained favor as a potential "window" on the neurobiology of schizophrenia. The variability in baseline concentrations and limitations in suppression of prolactin, however, represent inherent problems in using prolactin suppression as an indicator of dopamine receptor function (Powchik et al. 1987). Baseline prolactin levels are variable intraindividually and are affected by numerous factors, including gender, smoking, menstrual status, pregnancy, lactation, neuroleptic drugs, and the stress of hospitalization. Comparisons between groups are difficult when so many confounding factors need to be controlled. It is more meaningful to study the same individual at different states of illness (i.e., in relation to positive and negative symptoms and in relation to exacerbation and remission).

Baseline prolactin levels are increased, decreased, or not different in schizophrenic patients as compared to normal control subjects. Kleinman et al. (1982) found that prolactin levels vary inversely with Brief Psychiatric Rating Scale (BPRS) scores in schizophrenic patients with normal cerebral ventricles. Meltzer et al. (1983) confirmed this finding and showed an inverse relation between prolactin levels and delusions and hallucinations. These findings are consistent with the possibility that the increased dopamine function associated with positive symptoms is inversely related to prolactin secretion. This relation does not appear to be strong, however, and may be confined to females (Meltzer 1984).

Apomorphine, a direct dopamine agonist, reduces basal secretion of prolactin and has been used to challenge the dopamine system in schizophrenia. Prolactin suppression by apomorphine has been found to be blunted in schizophrenic patients (Davis et al. 1985; Rotrosen et al. 1979; Tamminga et al. 1977), but these studies were limited by their failure to control for such confounds as body weight, alcohol intake, and baseline prolactin levels. Meltzer and Busch (1986) showed an inverse correlation between severity of delusions and the prolactin response to chlorpromazine. Ferrier et al. (1983a) reported that prolactin response to thyrotropin-releasing hormone (TRH) was blunted in chronic schizophrenic patients who had been off drugs for more than a year, but Prange et al. (1979) failed to find such a difference. Clearly, there is no consensus to date, perhaps because of high variance in the measure, and no certainty about how prolactin levels might differ in patients with "negative" versus "positive" symptoms.

Growth Hormone

The regulation of growth hormone (GH) is complex. Many neurotransmitters, including dopamine, norepinephrine, acetylcholine, and serotonin, are involved in its release. Two peptides, GH-releasing factor and somatostatin, are also directly involved in its release. Other factors such as TRH, luteinizing hormone-releasing hormone, opioid peptides, sleep, hypoglycemia, stress, and exercise modulate GH release.

Baseline GH levels have not been found to differ significantly between schizophrenic and normal subjects (Lal 1987). In general, however, schizophrenic patients have more variable baseline GH secretion than normal controls (Cleghorn et al. 1983b; Kolakowska et al. 1981). Several agents have been used to stimulate GH release: insulin hypoglycemia, apomorphine, TRH, and sleep. Schizophrenic patients have been reported to have a reduced GH response to insulin hypoglycemia (Brambilla et al. 1975a). Brambilla et al. (1975a) also reported that reduced GH response to insulin was associated with negative symptoms such as negativism, asociality, and apathy, whereas increased GH release was associated with psychomotor excitement and hostility. The differences were attributed to possible differences in noradrenergic pathways mediating GH release in schizophrenic patients. Schimmelbusch et al. (1971) found a significantly reduced GH response to hypoglycemia in "back-ward" schizophrenic patients without, however, providing details about symptomatology. Chronic treatment-resistant "Kraepelinian" schizophrenic patients (defined as exhibiting defect state and deterioration) have also shown impaired GH response to glucose loading as compared to normal controls and non-Kraepelinian schizophrenic patients (Powchik et al. 1987).

Sleep-associated GH rise has been reported to be blunted in schizophrenic patients (Vigneri et al. 1974). In this study, one of the patients, an acute schizophrenic, had two clear GH rises during slow-wave sleep; the three chronic schizophrenic patients showed no increases in GH. GH release occurs principally in slow-wave sleep. Recent reports of an association between reduced slow-wave sleep and negative symptoms (Ganguli et al. 1987; Tandon et al. 1989a) provide further pilot support for a possible relationship between negative symptoms and GH release altered by slow-wave sleep.

Dopamine agonists have also been used to study the GH response in schizophrenic patients. In light of the dopamine hypothesis, one would anticipate that during psychotic exacerbations there would be an increased responsivity of GH to stimulation by dopamine agonists. This prediction has been confirmed in several studies, with acutely psychotic patients having enhanced GH responses to apomorphine (Cleghorn et al. 1983a; Muller-Spahn et al. 1984; Pandey et al. 1977; Whalley et al. 1984). Higher GH responses to apomorphine also have been noted in patients with elevated thought disorder scores (Zemlan et al. 1986a, 1986b). In particular, an association between Schneiderian first-rank symptoms and increased GH response to apomorphine has been noted (Whalley et al. 1984). On the other hand, a reduction in GH response to apomorphine has been observed in chronic schizophrenic patients (Ferrier et al. 1984; Pandey et al. 1977; Rotrosen et al. 1976). The possible confounding influence of age and body weight (chronic patients tending to be older and more obese) needs to be considered in interpreting such findings. A study involving young schizophrenic patients revealed an association between reduced GH responses to apomorphine and poor premorbid social functioning (Malas et al. 1987). Kleinman et al. (1982) and Ferrier et al. (1984) reported that the GH response to apomorphine was inversely related to negative symptoms in chronic schizophrenic patients. These findings provide some support for the hypothesis that dopaminergic hyperactivity is involved in the production of positive symptoms and decreased dopaminergic activity in the production of negative symptoms. Meltzer et al. (1986), however, actually noted a weak positive relation between GH response to apomorphine and negative symptoms.

TRH normally does not elicit GH release in humans. It can do so, however, in some patients with schizophrenia (DeMilio 1984; Ferrier et al. 1983a; Gil-Ad et al. 1981). TRH has significant effects on central nervous system receptors (Morley 1981) and enhances cholinergic function (Yarbrough 1979). Differential GH responses to TRH may therefore reflect differences in cholinergic activity between subgroups of schizophrenic patients. Keshavan et al. (1989b) examined the relationship between negative symptoms and the GH response to TRH in a sample of schizophrenic patients. A positive relationship was noted between Wing negative symptom scores (Wing 1961) and the baseline GH response to TRH. Negative symptom scores on the BPRS showed a trend toward a similar correlation with GH response to TRH ($r = .37$, $P = .07$). Positive symptom scores were not correlated significantly. Changes in the BPRS negative symptom scores after 3 to 4 weeks of treatment with haloperidol were related positively to the pretreatment GH response to TRH (Figure 8-1). GH response to TRH thus may be related to treatment-responsive negative symptoms in schizophrenia. GH response to TRH in humans appears to be mediated by muscarinic cholinergic receptors and is inhibited selectively by the muscarinic antagonist pirenzepine (Coiro et al. 1987). Tandon and Greden (1989) speculated that cholinergic hyperfunction may underlie the pathophysiology of negative symptoms. Our findings of a relationship between GH response to TRH and negative symptoms is consistent with the above hypothesis.

Clonidine, an alpha2-adrenergic agonist, releases GH. This response has been used as a test of central noradrenergic function (Lal et al. 1975). Lal et al. (1983) failed to observe significant differences between schizophrenic and normal subjects in clonidine-induced GH release, although schizophrenic subjects showed a greater variability in the GH response. Muller-Spahn et al. (1986), however, reported that the GH response to clonidine was significantly lower in chronic schizophrenic patients in whom the dominant symptoms were affective flattening, lack of interest, and anergia. It should be noted that 5 of the 17 patients also had florid symptoms such as delusions and hallucinations. The authors speculated that "minus" symptoms were related to impaired central noradrenergic function.

Gonadal Hormones

Early studies using testicular biopsies and urinary testosterone levels showed some reductions in gonadal function in schizophrenia (Hemphill et al. 1944; Hoskins and Pincus 1949). Basal levels of follicle-stimulating hormone and luteinizing hormone have been found to be lower in schizophrenic patients than in controls (Brambilla et al. 1976). More recent studies have shown a lower frequency of secretory episodes of luteinizing hormone and follicle-stimulating

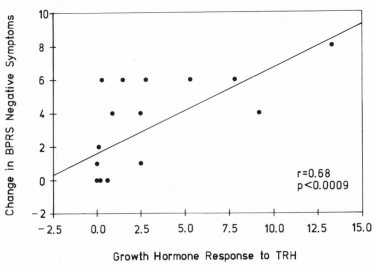

Figure 8-1. Thyrotropin-releasing hormone (TRH)-induced growth hormone response and negative symptom change with neuroleptic treatment in 20 patients. BPRS = Brief Psychiatric Rating Scale.

hormone in chronic schizophrenic patients (Ferrier et al. 1982). An inverse relation has been found between the extent of positive symptoms and follicle-stimulating hormone (Ferrier et al. 1982; Johnstone et al. 1977); no such relation was noticed with negative symptoms. Dopamine infusion reduces luteinizing hormone levels and the number of luteinizing hormone secretory episodes (Huseman et al. 1980), and neuroleptics reverse the gonadotropic abnormalities in schizophrenic patients (Brambilla et al. 1975b). Based on these observations, Crow et al. (1986) speculated that the depression in gonadotropin levels and its relation to positive symptoms may be related to increased dopaminergic function. Dopamine, however, has been shown to stimulate as well as to inhibit gonadotropin-releasing hormone from human hypothalami in vitro (Rasmussen et al. 1986), making any meaningful interpretation of these findings difficult.

Responses of gonadotropic hormones to releasing hormone stimulation have also been reported to be abnormal in schizophrenic patients (Brambilla 1980). Whether these alterations bear a relation to positive or negative symptom complexes remains unclear.

Hypothalamic-Pituitary-Adrenal Axis

The Type II schizophrenia syndrome with negative symptoms and cognitive impairment was found to be associated with elevated postdexamethasone cortisol levels (Coppen et al. 1983; Harris 1985; Saffer et al. 1985). There is some evidence for a relationship among negative symptoms, tardive dyskinesia, and cognitive impairment in schizophrenia (Crow 1980a; Sorokin et al. 1988). Crow suggested that negative symptoms may be related to structural abnormalities in the brains of schizophrenic patients. Keshavan et al. (1989a) have also observed an association between dexamethasone nonsuppression and cerebral ventricular enlargement in schizophrenia. This supposition is supported by observations that dexamethasone suppression test results are frequently abnormal in dementia (Coryell 1984). A review of the literature reveals widely discrepant rates of dexamethasone nonsuppression in schizophrenia and inconsistencies regarding the association of this finding with negative symptoms. Variable medication status and phase of illness at least partially explain these anomalies. Higher rates of dexamethasone nonsuppression are generally noted in medication-free patients during an acute exacerbation than in neuroleptic-stabilized chronic schizophrenic patients. Moreover, several investigations (Baumgartner et al. 1986; Moller et al. 1986; Wik et al. 1986) have noted high rates of dexamethasone nonsuppression in the acute phase of schizophrenic illness with normalization following resolution of acute symptoms. Tandon et al. (1989d) and Mazzara et al. (1989) reported similar findings and noted an association between negative symptoms and postdexa-methasone cortisol levels only at medication-free baseline but not after 4 weeks following neuroleptic treatment. Keshavan et al. (1989a) failed to observe such an association, possibly because of differences in patient samples (Tandon et al. 1989b). Tandon and Greden (1989) speculated that negative symptoms in schizophrenia may be related to cholinergic hyperfunction, particularly in the acute psychotic phase of the illness. Since cholinergic agonists stimulate corticotropin-releasing hormone secretion in the hypothalamic-pituitary-adrenal axis (Carroll et al. 1980; Toumisto and Mannisto 1985), it is possible that cholinergic hyperfunction may underlie both negative symptoms and dexamethasone nonsuppression in the acute phase of schizophrenia. The relationship between dexamethasone suppression test findings and clinical features in schizoprenia is reviewed in detail by Tandon et al. (1990d).

Hypothalamic-Pituitary-Thyroid Axis

Interest in this area began with the observation of Gjessing and Gjessing (1961) that thyroid hormones are efficacious in the treat-ment of periodic catatonia. The literature on thyroid indices in schizophrenia, however, is conflicting. Thyrotropin-stimulating hor-mone response to TRH has been reported to be impaired in about one-third of patients with schizophrenia and schizoaffective disorder (Langer et al. 1984, 1986; Wolkin et al. 1984), although other investigators do not agree (Loosen 1985). Targum (1983) and Langer et al. (1986) reported that abnormal TRH tests predict an episodic illness with better prognosis in patients with schizo-phreniform disorder and schizophrenia. It is thus possible that abnor-mal (blunted) thyrotropin-stimulating hormone responses to TRH may be related to psychopathologic syndromes with differing prog-noses. The relation between TRH tests and the positive-negative syndromes has not been investigated.

Posterior Pituitary

A significant percentage (6–17%) of chronic psychiatric patients have polydipsia and polyuria without identifiable medical cause, with 69–83% of such patients being schizophrenic (Illowski and Kirch 1988). A possible hypothalamic defect involving an inappropriate secretion of antidiuretic hormone is the most likely pathophysiologic mechanism (Hobson and English 1963). Vieweg et al. (1985) sug-gested that this complication occurs in the "preterminal" phase of schizophrenia, characterized by Arieti (1945) as manifesting disor-ganization, lack of emotional content, and compulsive behavior. Kirch et al. (1985) reported enlarged cerebral ventricle and intellectual decline (a clinical description conforming to the description of "Type II" schizophrenia advanced by Crow 1980a) in the majority of schizophrenic patients with polydipsia and hyponatremia. The number of patients studied is too small to draw firm conclusions. Any future assessments of vasopressin and oxytocin in schizophrenic patients should seek to compare those with predominantly positive and negative symptoms.

Miscellaneous Peptides

Several peptides have been implicated in the pathophysiology of schizophrenia. Roberts et al. (1983) examined the regional distribution of peptides in schizophrenic patients categorized as Type I (mainly positive symptoms) or Type II (mainly negative symptoms). Cholecystokinin was lower in the hippocampus of Type II patients and in the temporal cortex of both Type I and Type II as compared to normal controls; Type I patients had elevated levels of vasoactive intestinal peptide in the amygdala. Hippocampal substance P was elevated in both types. They speculated that the increase in vasoactive intestinal peptide could be a consequence of altered dopamine input to the lateral amygdala and that the reductions in cholecystokinin in Type II patients may be unrelated to dopaminergic alterations. These findings have not been confirmed in more recent studies.

CONCLUSIONS

The neuroendocrine research strategy has so far shed little light on the pathophysiology of schizophrenia; one of the main reasons for this failure may be the heterogeneity of schizophrenia. This review suggests that there may be some neuroendocrine differences between subgroups of schizophrenia as defined by positive and negative symptoms, but that the following caveats are in order. First, interpretation of neuroendocrine studies in schizophrenia requires careful consideration of "confounding" variables that may affect neuroendocrine function: the effects of prior neuroleptic therapy, sex, age, time of the day, physical exercise, luteal phase, body weight, intercurrent illness, and emotional state. Second, the neuroendocrine control of pituitary hormone responses to various kinds of stimulation is exceedingly complex, with multiple neurotransmitters being involved. Third, the assumption underlying pituitary hormone studies in schizophrenia is that abnormalities in tuberoinfundibular pituitary function reflect similar alterations in the mesolimbic system; however, this assumption is unproven. Finally, several problems still beset the identification and definition of positive and negative symptoms as described in other chapters. Problems in relating positive and negative symptoms to central nervous system dysfunction include the cross-sectional concurrence of these two symptom dimensions and the change of symptoms over time.

Although the above considerations mandate caution in interpreting the literature, some trends are worthy of further attention (Table 8-1). First, weak evidence exists for an inverse relation between basal prolactin levels and positive symptoms. Blunted GH responses to

Table 8-1. Positive and negative symptoms in schizophrenia: associations with neuroendocrine findings

Variable	Symptoms	
	Positive	Negative
Growth hormone	Associated with increased growth hormone response to apomorphine	Associated with increased growth hormone response to TRH, and possibly with reduced growth hormone release to clonidine, hypoglycemia, apomorphine, and sleep
Prolactin	Weekly associated inversely with baseline, and TRH-stimulated prolactin secretion	
Gonadotropins	Inverse relation between FSH and positive symptoms	
Pituitary-adrenal axis		Dexamethasone non-suppression related to cerebral ventricular enlargement and probably to negative symptoms
Vasopressin		SIADH possibly more frequent in "defect" state schizophrenic patients
Miscellaneous peptides	Increased in vaspactive intestinal peptide in amygdala; increased hippocampal substance P - ??	Reduced cholecystokinin in hippocampus; increased hippocampal substance P - ??

Note. TRH = thyrotropin-releasing hormone. FSH = follicle-stimulating hormone. SIADH = syndrome of inappropriate secretion of antidiuretic hormone.

apomorphine, and possibly clonidine, hypoglycemia, and sleep, seem to be related to defect symptoms, while enhanced GH release in response to apomorphine may correlate with positive symptoms. Enhanced GH response to TRH, dexamethasone nonsuppression, and aberrant gonadotropin responses may be associated with negative symptoms and with such other features of the schizophrenic defect state as ventricular enlargement and cognitive impairment. The tendency to polydipsia and hyponatremia frequently seen in schizophrenia also appears to be related to features of the schizophrenic defect state. The relation of other neuroendocrine parameters to symptomatic subtypes within schizophrenia remains unclear.

The neurotransmitter correlates of the observed neuroendocrine dysregulation in schizophrenia may provide clues to the pathophysiology of positive and negative syndromes. The association between blunted apomorphine-induced GH response and negative symptoms is consistent with the possibility of deficient dopamine function in the negative syndrome (Friedhoff 1986; Mackay 1980; Meltzer 1986; van Kammen et al. 1986b). Enhanced GH responses to apomorphine, abnormalities in gonadotropin levels, and low prolactin levels in relation to positive symptoms is similarly consistent with possible dopamine hyperfunction in the mediation of such symptoms (Crow 1980b).

Insulin-induced hypoglycemia seems to stimulate a noradrenergically mediated GH release. Blunted GH responses to hypoglycemia as well as to clonidine in patients with the schizophrenic defect state may thus point to impaired noradrenergic mechanisms in the negative syndrome. Cholinergic mechanisms are predominantly involved in adrenocorticotropin hormone release (Toumisto and Mannisto 1985). The observed associations between negative symptoms, dexamethasone nonsuppression and enhanced GH release by TRH are consistent with the possibility of cholinergic hyperfunction in such patients.

In summary, the neuroendocrine strategy may be useful in validating the positive and negative symptom dimensions in schizophrenia, but no clear consensus findings have emerged to date. Although such symptoms do not appear to be directly caused by or related to endocrine abnormalities, the neuroendocrine strategy could be useful in providing concurrent validity or in evaluating the relationship of various neurotransmitters to these symptoms. For this purpose, use of neuroendocrine perturbation tests involving more selective neurotransmitter agonists or antagonists would be desirable. Further studies should also incorporate well-characterized patients, well-studied controls, a longitudinal approach, and careful consideration of the methodological issues addressed in this chapter.

Structural and Developmental Theories

Chapter 9

CT and MRI Abnormalities in Schizophrenia: Relationship With Negative Symptoms

Stephen C. Olson, M.D.
Henry A. Nasrallah, M.D.
Jeffrey A. Coffman, M.D.
Steven B. Schwarzkopf, M.D.

Chapter 9

CT and MRI Abnormalities in Schizophrenia: Relationship With Negative Symptoms

> Dilatation of the ventricles (hydrocephalus chronicus) is frequently found in the insane...[Regarding chronic insanity] between partial dementia and dementia there is as little difference, anatomically, as between melancholia and mania: still, generally speaking, considerable atrophy of the brain corresponds to a condition of profound mental weakness. (The reverse, however, does not hold good.)
>
> —Griesinger (1882)

The above words should humble the modern psychiatric researcher investigating the relationship between brain morphology and the phenomenology of psychosis, considering that they were written in the late 1800s. Much of what we consider essential to scientific study of the subject—diagnostic criteria, statistical method, brain imaging—was not even conceptualized at the time. Wilhelm Griesinger was clearly a pioneer in neuropsychiatry and helped establish the concept of mental illness as a disease of the brain. The terminology is dated, of course, but the question of brain atrophy in dementia (schizophrenia) and its relation to profound mental weakness (the deficit syndrome) is very much alive.

For a century after Griesinger, neuroscientists struggled with the only methods then available—postmortem neuropathology and pneumoencephalography—to confirm the association between ventriculomegaly and schizophrenic defect (Cazzullo 1963; Huber 1957; Jacobi and Winkler 1927). Methodological limitations inherent in both techniques made large-scale study of the gross neuroanatomy of schizophrenia unfeasible until the advent of noninvasive neuroimaging in the 1970s. In this chapter, we will be concerned with the results of studies utilizing X-ray computed tomography (CT) and, more recently, magnetic resonance imaging (MRI) that have addressed the relationship of brain morphology to the deficit syndrome or negative symptoms in schizophrenia.

CT SCAN STUDIES

A comprehensive review of CT studies of schizophrenia (Shelton and Weinberger 1986) reported that 26 of 35 studies showed statistically significant lateral ventricular enlargement in schizophrenia compared to nonpsychiatric controls. The ventricle-brain ratio (VBR) is the most widely used index of ventricular enlargement and is calculated by dividing the area of the lateral ventricles by the area of the brain in the same cut. Other consistent findings include sulcal widening (14 of 20 studies positive), third ventricular enlargement (10 of 12 studies), and cerebellar atrophy. Much less certain are scattered reports of reversed cerebral asymmetry and CT density alterations. The relationship of anatomic abnormalities other than lateral ventricular enlargement to negative symptomatology has been relatively unexplored.

The initial report of increased ventricular size by CT in chronic schizophrenic patients by Johnstone et al. (1976) also confronted the association of ventriculomegaly with the defect state. The authors studied 18 male long-stay patients (duration of hospitalization, 20–42 years) meeting Feighner's criteria (Feighner et al. 1972) for schizophrenia. The patient group had significantly enlarged lateral ventricles relative to a control group ($P < .01$), with almost no overlap between the two groups. Moreover, the degree of ventricular enlargement was highly correlated with the severity of cognitive impairment on the Withers-Hinton scale (Withers and Hinton 1971). Also noted were nonsignificant correlations between ventricular size and positive features ($r = -.24$) and negative features ($r = +.38$) in the 13 subjects who had not undergone a leukotomy. The report of this study emphasized the issues that have continued to be central to a critical review of this topic: subject and control selection (Raz et al. 1988; Smith and Iacono 1988) and method of measurement (Zatz and Jernigan 1983).

Although not specifically addressing the deficit state, the first studies in the United States showed a high rate of ventriculomegaly in schizophrenic patients and that the subgroup with large ventricles had features associated with a more severe illness: poor premorbid adjustment (Weinberger et al. 1980b) and poor response to treatment (Weinberger et al. 1980a).

The lengthy hospitalizations and severe cognitive impairment of schizophrenic subjects in the Johnstone et al. (1976) study limit its generalizability to the general population of schizophrenic patients. However, the extreme degree of ventricular enlargement and the severe cognitive impairment seen in these subjects supports the inference that, within the whole of schizophrenia, these phenomena are linked. This view was supported in an early study (Donnelly et al. 1980) of a small group of young chronic schizophrenic patients in whom CT abnormality was correctly predicted in 80% of subjects by impairment on the Halstead-Reitan Neuropsychological Test Battery (Reitan 1979). More recent investigations of the link between increased VBR and Halstead-Reitan battery impairment have concluded that schizophrenic patients perform in the brain-damaged range on cognitive tests due to an intrinsic dementing process; in severe cases, this deficit is associated with structural abnormalities (Lawson et al. 1988). Negative reports have employed less comprehensive batteries of neuropsychological tests (Obiols et al. 1987; Rossi et al. 1987).

The first systematic study (Andreasen et al. 1982) of the association of increased VBR and negative symptoms (Andreasen 1982) is widely cited as indicating an association between ventricular enlargement and a preponderance of negative symptoms. From a group of 52 subjects meeting DSM-III (American Psychiatric Association 1980) criteria and Research Diagnostic Criteria (RDC) (Spitzer et al. 1978) for schizophrenia, 16 with VBR > 1 SD above the control mean were compared with the 16 schizophrenic subjects with the smallest VBR on the Scale for the Assessment of Positive Symptoms (SAPS) (Andreasen 1984) and the Scale for the Assessment of Negative Symptoms (SANS) (Andreasen 1983) at the time of admission to the hospital. Large VBR patients had significantly lower cognitive function and ratings of positive symptoms, especially bizarre behavior, and tended to have higher negative symptoms. Finally, consistent with the authors' conception of a bipolar relationship between positive and negative symptoms, a positive minus negative score was calculated, which was more negative (less positive) in the large VBR group. Since the negative symptom ratings were done at the time of admission and may reflect a process distinct from the residual deficit state (reviewed in Chapters 1, 2, and 4 of this volume), this report may be more narrowly interpreted as linking small ventricles with more severe positive symptoms than the converse. In another analysis of the same sample (Andreasen and Olsen 1982), the patients were separated by predominance of symptom type into negative, positive, and mixed schizophrenia. A significantly larger VBR was found in the negative schizophrenia group, which also had more unemployment and higher ratings of premorbid sociosexual dysfunction.

Comparable findings (more positive symptoms in small VBR subjects compared to a large VBR group) have also been reported in drug-free schizophrenic patients (Luchins et al. 1984). Negative symptoms were nonsignificantly greater in the schizophrenic patients with small VBR, the opposite direction from that reported by Andreasen et al. (1982). Notably, the largest VBR group did not show improvement after 5 weeks of neuroleptic treatment in contrast to the rest of the patients. There was no difference in overall positive or negative symptom change during the drug treatment, but analysis of individual items indicated a deterioration in paranoid delusions, psychomotor retardation, and bizarre behavior in the three patients with VBR > 2 SD above the control mean.

According to Pearlson et al. (1984), persistently unemployed patients with either schizophrenia or bipolar disorder had larger VBR than employed patients or controls, suggesting that this relationship may not be specific to schizophrenia. Also, a correlation between VBR and negative symptoms was found in both patient groups, and negative symptoms tended to be higher in the group with VBR > 1 SD above the control mean. Other features associated with increased VBR in this sample were earlier onset and poorer premorbid adjustment (Pearlson et al. 1985).

In contrast to the above reports finding both cognitive impairment and increased negative symptoms in large VBR groups, other investigations have shown an association of none or only one of these indicators of the deficit state with ventricular enlargement. Two studies revealed cognitive dysfunction but no difference in clinical symptoms in patients with large ventricles (Nasrallah et al. 1983b; Pandurangi et al. 1986). These studies used a similar research design, comparing a subgroup of male schizophrenic patients above a cutoff defined by the control VBR to the remainder of the schizophrenic sample. Nasrallah et al. observed a nonsignificantly higher rate of impairment on the Mini-Mental State Exam (Folstein et al. 1975), and Pandurangi et al. found more impairment on Halstead-Reitan impairment indices in the high VBR group. Both studies tallied the presence or absence of various positive and negative symptoms and found no differences in the frequency of any particular symptom between groups, nor any difference in rating of premorbid function. When the Nasrallah et al. sample was divided on the basis of cortical sulcal widening, the group with sulcal widening was found to have less agitation and more Mini-Mental State Exam impairment than the group with normal sulci (Nasrallah et al. 1983a). VBR was no greater in the sulcal widening group, supporting the notion of independent pathoplastic processes responsible for these morphological differences (Nasrallah et al. 1982; Weinberger et al. 1979).

In a more recent study, Pandurangi et al. (1988) were able to replicate several findings linking CT abnormalities to various indicators of deterioration. Thirty-two hospitalized subjects were evaluated with the Premorbid Adjustment Scale of Cannon-Spoor et al. (1982) and with positive and negative symptoms ratings. The authors conceptualized the ratings of positive and negative symptoms as reflecting "state and trait aspects of psychopathology," respectively, and consequently rated positive symptoms for the worst week preceding the evaluation, but rated negative symptoms for a more extended period of time, excluding the acute episode. Subjects were divided into groups with ventricular enlargement only, sulcal widening only, or both findings. In the whole sample, VBR was negatively correlated with premorbid adjustment and a thought disorder factor derived from the symptom ratings; sulcal widening was associated with indices of social deterioration. Patients with abnormal CTs displayed fewer positive symptoms, especially those loading on the thought disorder factor. No relation to negative symptoms was observed. Sulcal widening seemed to indicate a more malignant disease process, with those subjects having somewhat better premorbid function but more current negative symptoms. Cortical atrophy, present in 33% of schizophrenic patients in another study (Vita et al. 1988), was more frequent in males and related to duration of illness and ventricular enlargement, but not to Wechsler Adult Intelligence Scale (Wechsler 1981) performance, occupational impairment, DSM-III subtype, or clinical response to neuroleptics.

Owens et al. (1985) reported a large, well-designed study of ventricular size and its correlates in a total of 192 subjects, mostly schizophrenic inpatients (n =110) compared to smaller samples of schizophrenic outpatients, bipolar patients, and a control group of neurotic patients. The schizophrenic inpatients were selected from a larger group of 510 patients studied previously (Owens and Johnstone 1980) to provide matched subsamples to address various research questions. One hypothesis tested was whether schizophrenic patients with the "defect state"—as defined by prominent affective flattening, poverty of speech, and cognitive impairment—had larger ventricles than an age-, sex-, treatment-, and education-matched comparison group. Seven matched pairs with and without the defect syndrome did not differ on VBR; similar groups matched for presence versus absence of deteriorating course, educational attainment, or catatonic syndrome did not differ on VBR.

Based on a highly significant correlation of VBR and increasing age, the sample was divided into five ranges of age-corrected VBR based on the mean ±SD of the neurotic group. An inverted U-shaped relationship was found between ventricular size and cognitive function, with greater frequency of marked impairment at both large and small extremes of VBR. A significant positive correlation between VBR and impairment of social behavior and activity was noted. The only positive or negative symptom from the Krawiecka scale (Krawiecka et al. 1977) that related to VBR was hallucinations; these were less frequent in the highest VBR category (mean +2). Finally, a strong association between ventricular size and involuntary movement disorder, which the authors link to schizophrenic deterioration, was observed.

Kemali et al. (1985, 1987) confirmed many of the reported associations between structural brain abnormalities and defect symptomatology in an investigation of subjects meeting DSM-III schizophrenia criteria compared to age-, sex-, and education-matched controls. Duration of illness and time hospitalized distinguished the large VBR schizophrenic patients from the rest of the sample. This abnormal CT group also had higher ratings of alogia, affective flattening, and attentional impairment on the SANS, poorer ratings of self-care, and more impaired performance on a variety of neuropsychological measures.

Other studies of the interrelationships of negative symptoms, cognitive impairment, and ventricular enlargement (Keilp et al. 1988; Losonczy et al. 1986a, 1986b) have failed to replicate the early observations of Johnstone et al. (1976) and Andreasen and Olsen (1982). Losonczy et al. found no relationship between VBR, response to a controlled trial of haloperidol, and positive or negative symptoms. The authors identified a subgroup of "Kraepelinian" schizophrenic patients who were chronically unemployed and dependent on others for provision of necessities of living; this extremely impaired sample had asymmetric lateral ventricles that were 28% larger on the left. In the Keilp et al. (1988) study, acute and chronic, but not subacute or subchronic, RDC schizophrenic patients had larger VBRs than did the control subjects. Possible interaction between duration of illness and response to treatment, which may have confounded the relationship of VBR and symptom change, were not reported. Another group found no relation of VBR to admission Brief Psychiatric Rating Scale (Overall and Gorham 1962) scores, but at discharge, VBR was negatively correlated with depression, tension, and blunted affect (Bishop et al. 1983).

Gender differences in VBR in controls and schizophrenic patients have usually not emerged (Cazzullo et al. 1989; Owens et al. 1985; Pearlson et al. 1985) when females have been included in CT studies. However, two studies (Shelton et al. 1988; Williams et al. 1985) suggest that sex differences must be considered in interpretation of cerebral morphology, at least in some samples. Shelton et al. observed that while lateral ventricular size and ratings of sulcal markings did not reveal gender-related differences, third ventricle width differed more between control and schizophrenic females than between the male samples.

Williams et al. (1985) also found gender-dependent morphological differences, comparing stable neuroleptic-treated RDC schizophrenic and schizoaffective patients to age-matched controls. A trend (.10 > P > .05) was noted for VBR to be greater in males in both the schizophrenic and normal groups. When the VBR values for controls were pooled and an enlarged ventricle group of schizophrenic patients was selected based on a cutoff of 1 SD above the control mean, 12 of 13 were male, compared to the total schizophrenic sample, in which 30 of 40 were male. Consequently, the large VBR group was identified with separate cutoff scores for males and females. This large VBR group was more likely to meet criteria for schizophrenia and had worse outcome, more chronic negative symptoms, and more premorbid psychosocial impairment. When schizoaffective patients were excluded (all were in the normal VBR group), only the outcome measure remained significant, although trends were apparent in the other clinical deficit state markers. Exclusion of good-outcome patients from the comparison of large and small VBR groups rendered all clinical differences nonsignificant. Subtle neurologic dysfunction, intellectual impairment, age, family history, duration of illness, and early childhood cerebral insult did not differ between the large and normal VBR groups. The authors concluded that ventricular enlargement is related to a subtype of schizophrenia with unfavorable outcome, rather than an etiologically distinct "organic" subtype.

MRI STUDIES

Only four studies utilizing MRI that address the clinical correlates of the deficit state have been published. Besson et al. (1987) found that ventricular enlargement was associated with age and duration of illness, with a trend toward higher negative symptom ratings. Differences between small subgroups divided on the basis of positive and negative symptoms indicated differences in the T1 relaxation time between groups in discrete brain regions, but there were no differences between the schizophrenic groups and controls. Due to the small sample and methodological concerns over the reliability of measurement of MRI tissue parameters, these results await further exploration and replication.

In another study (Mathew et al. 1985), midsagittal MRI was used to measure the area of the corpus callosum and the septum pellucidum, which was employed as a measure of the midsagittal extent of the lateral ventricles. Septal areas were related to age, but neither callosal nor septal areas were correlated with total positive or negative symptoms. Another MRI study focused on the corpus callosum in male schizophrenic patients and controls and found a larger anterior callosum in schizophrenia (Uematsu and Kaiya 1988). A variety of demographic and clinical variables were studied in relation to several callosal measures; generally enlargement of the corpus callosum was associated with poorer heterosexual relations, fewer hospitalizations, and lower educational attainment.

The first extensive study of schizophrenia using MRI was that of Andreasen et al. (1986). This group found smaller midsagittal areas of the cranium, cerebrum, and frontal region in schizophrenic males, implicating an early developmental process interfering with the normal growth of the brain. In males, six of nine subjects with the smallest cranial areas had prominent negative symptoms, compared to zero of nine with the largest cranial areas. A similar relationship was observed for cerebral but not frontal size. Cognitive test scores of frontal function and visual memory significantly predicted cranial size corrected for sex and height, indicating poorer cognitive function in patients with smaller crania. A recent MRI study from this group (Andreasen et al. 1990a) could not replicate these findings of decreased frontal, cerebral, and cranial size in schizophrenic patients. A prominent sex effect was observed in this study, with male patients showing most of the increase in ventricular size. This study also noted a significant relationship between negative symptoms and ventricular size.

In summary, an extensive literature on the relation of ventricular enlargement and sulcal widening to indicators of the deficit syndrome, particularly cognitive impairment, negative symptoms, and response to neuroleptic treatment, does not consistently confirm an association between these factors. Synthesis of the findings will be discussed below, but at present it cannot be determined with certainty as to whether morphological differences are indicative of a subgroup with poor outcome, an "organic" subtype of schizophrenia, both of the above, or neither. Other abnormalities such as third ventricle enlargement, decreased brain size, callosal size, and MRI parameters have been reported too infrequently to draw any conclusions at this time as to their relation to deficit symptoms.

The Ohio State University MRI Study

We are currently addressing many of the research questions raised by the literature on brain morphology and its relation to clinical manifestations of major psychoses in the Schizophrenia Research Program at The Ohio State University. The methodology includes a comprehensive study of brain structure as assessed by MRI, brain function by computerized electroencephalogram and evoked potential mapping, extensive neuropsychological testing, and clinical and etiologic assessments. We will present here results bearing on the relation of structural abnormalities in the ventricular system to positive and negative symptoms in clinically stable, treated subjects with schizophrenia or schizoaffective disorder.

Subjects to date were recruited from clinical settings at The Ohio State University Hospitals and through local practitioners and family advocacy groups. Diagnoses were made by psychiatrists based on all available data including structured interview (Structured Clinical Interview for DSM-III-R [Spitzer et al. 1986]), informant reports, and medical records. Subjects met DSM-III-R (American Psychiatric Association 1987) criteria for schizophrenia or schizoaffective disorder, were 18–50 years of age, gave informed consent, and were excluded for significant substance abuse, neurologic disease, head injury with loss of consciousness, or metallic implants.

MRIs were acquired using a GE 1.5 tesla MRI system with inversion recovery imaging parameters. The images were projected to approximately two times life size and the margins of brain structures outlined and measured with a computerized digital tablet. Measurements of the lateral ventricles and cerebral area were made on two cuts, one in the midsagittal plane and one in the coronal plane in the slice immediately posterior to the optic chiasm. The correlation between midsagittal and coronal VBR measures was 0.775 ($P <$ .0001). All prior studies of ventricular enlargement have either measured the VBR in the transverse plane or calculated a volumetric estimate of ventricular size. In order to construct a VBR which more closely approximates a volumetric estimate, the VBRs in the midsagittal and coronal planes were averaged to create a two-plane VBR.

Patients were assessed on the SANS and the SAPS for determination of negative and positive symptoms, done at the time of discharge for the small proportion of subjects who were recruited from the inpatient service. Global ratings (range, 0–5) on the five categories on each scale were used in the analysis. Principal components analysis of the 10 global ratings was performed in the 75 subjects with complete SANS and SAPS ratings. The item weighting of the three Varimax orthogonal factors is shown in Table 9-1. Inspection of the table reveals that the first factor is predominately loaded on negative symptoms, the second on delusions and hallucinations, and the third on features of disorganization, similar to the formal thought disorder factor identified by others (Liddle 1987a; Pandurangi et al. 1988). These three factors are hereafter referred to as the negative symptom, delusion-hallucination, and disorganization factors.

Inspection of the VBR distribution revealed a bimodal distribution, with 11 subjects falling above a cutoff of 6.5%, 8 of whom were male schizophrenic patients. Compared to the remaining 64 subjects, the high VBR group tended to be older (mean age 35.4 versus 31.1 years, two-tailed t test, P = .054) and to have lower scores on the disorganization factor (mean -0.49 versus 0.09, P = .073). The groups did not differ on negative or delusion-hallucination factors, age at first hospitalization, or education.

Two-way analyses of variance to investigate gender, diagnosis, or interaction effects on VBR and the SANS and SAPS factors were performed. Significant results shown in Tables 9-2 and 9-3 demonstrate that males tend to have higher ratings on the negative symptom factor and that schizophrenic subjects have larger ventricles than schizoaffective subjects. This suggested that grouping all subjects together in the analysis might obscure relationships between ventricular enlargement and clinical ratings; consequently, male schizophrenic subjects were examined separately in the following analyses.

Table 9-1. Orthogonal factor structure for SANS and SAPS global ratings (N = 75)

	Factor 1	Factor 2	Factor 3
Affective flattening	.828	−.069	.162
Alogia	.794	−.148	.33
Avolition	.782	.167	.134
Anhedonia	.819	.223	.011
Attentional impairment	.49	−.102	.666
Hallucinations	−.006	.856	.1
Delusions	.11	.838	.208
Bizarre behavior	.041	.261	.793
Positive formal thought	.157	.173	.73
Variance explained	.398	.192	.114

Note. SANS = Scale for the Assessment of Negative Symptoms. SAPS = Scale for the Assessment of Positive Symptoms.

The eight subjects with VBR > 6.5% were compared with the 33 male schizophrenic subjects below that cutoff on the SANS and SAPS factors; the same pattern as noted in the entire sample was observed: no difference in negative and delusion-hallucination factors and a trend for lower thought disorder in the large VBR group ($P = .08$). Age, onset, and duration of illness did not differ in the two groups.

The 41 male schizophrenic subjects were divided into upper and lower VBR groups by dividing at the median VBR of 4.27%. The two groups were compared by t test on age, onset, duration and SANS and SAPS factors and by Mann-Whitney U for individual SANS and SAPS items, which were non-normally distributed. The upper VBR group had higher negative symptom factor scores and were more impaired on the affective flattening, alogia, and anhedonia items from the SANS (Table 9-4). Examination of the same clinical variables in the upper and lower VBR quartiles ($n = 10$ in each quartile) showed the same magnitude of association, but none of the comparisons reached statistical significance due to the small sample sizes. Non-parametric correlation of VBR with these measures was significant for

Table 9-2. Sex and diagnosis effects on negative symptom factor

	Male	Female
Schizoaffective	.22 ± 1.17	−.38 ± 1.08
	$n = 13$	$n = 8$
Schizophrenia	.11 ± 1.01	−.35 ± .60
	$n = 41$	$n = 13$
Source	F test	P value
Diagnosis	.01918	.8902
Sex	3.78065	.0558
Diagnosis × sex	.06561	.7986

Table 9-3. Sex and diagnosis effects on ventricle-brain ratio

	Male	Female
Schizoaffective	3.91 ± 1.42	3.57 ± 1.40
	$n = 13$	$n = 8$
Schizophrenia	4.57 ± 1.82	4.93 ± 1.94
	$n = 42$	$n = 15$
Source	F test	P value
Diagnosis	4.56124	.036
Sex	.0004	.9841
Diagnosis × sex	.55658	.458

the negative symptom factor (Spearman rho = .38, P = .022, two-tailed) and alogia (rho = .35, P = .03) and approached significance for affective flattening (rho = .30, P = .07) and anhedonia (rho = .31, P = .06).

DISCUSSION

Our study confirms a relationship in chronic psychoses between lateral ventricular size, as measured by the mean of the VBRs in the coronal and midsagittal planes, and more severe negative symptoms, particularly in schizophrenic males. This association was evident whether subjects were divided into two groups at the median or at a high cutoff that identifies a subgroup with ventricles above the normal range, or whether clinical measures were correlated with VBR across the entire range of subjects. This would tend to argue against a subtype of schizophrenia characterized by ventriculomegaly and prominent deficit state, but rather suggests that some dysplastic or atrophic process is associated with the severity of deficit symptoms. It cannot be assumed that the brain structural abnormality is of primary

Table 9-4. SANS and SAPS ratings and illness variables for schizophrenic males

Variable	Upper VBR (>4.25%) n = 20	Lower VBR (<4.25%) n = 21	P
Age	32.8 ± 6.5	30.3 ± 6.1	NS
Age first hospitalization	23.0 ± 5.6	21.8 ± 4.7	NS
Duration of illness	10.3 ± 5.7	9.2 ± 5.3	NS
SANS/SAPS factors			
Negative symptoms	0.50 ± .94	−0.26 ± .96	.015
Delusion/hallucination	0.08 ± 1.15	0.05 ± 1.02	NS
Disorganization	−0.05 ± 1.24	0.18 ± 1.24	NS
SANS global items			
Affective flattening	2.5 ± 1.5	1.6 ± 1.4	.052
Alogia	2.3 ± 1.6	1.2 ± 1.3	.023
Avolition	2.5 ± 1.4	2.3 ± 1.5	NS
Anhedonia	3.3 ± 1.4	2.1 ± 1.5	.019
Attentional impairment	2.0 ± 1.8	1.4 ± 1.4	NS
SAPS global items			
Hallucinations	2.0 ± 1.9	2.0 ± 1.8	NS
Delusions	2.3 ± 1.7	2.0 ± 1.8	NS
Bizarre behavior	0.5 ± 1.0	0.9 ± 1.3	NS
Positive thought disorder	1.4 ± 1.8	1.5 ± 1.6	NS

Note. SANS = Scale for the Assessment of Negative Symptoms. SAPS = Scale for the Assessment of Positive Symptoms. VBR = ventricle-brain ratio.

etiologic significance to the development of negative symptoms; both findings could be secondary to a common pathophysiologic factor.

The vast majority of subjects in our study were stable outpatients living in the community and more typical of the severely mentally disabled population served by private and community mental health center practitioners than the long-term hospital population sampled in some other studies. Our sample appears closest in composition to that studied by Williams et al. (1985), who also found male schizophrenic patients overrepresented in the large VBR group. Relationships between VBR and negative symptoms seen in this study in male schizophrenic subjects were absent in female subjects. Whether this is due to the trend for lower negative symptoms in females in our sample, the greater sensitivity to or frequency of brain insult in males (Nasrallah and Wilcox 1989), or gender differences in outcome and response to treatment cannot be determined at this time.

The awareness that negative symptoms seen in acute exacerbations of schizophrenia respond to neuroleptic treatment (Goldberg 1985) and may reflect different physiologic processes than the persistent deficit syndrome has important implications for the study of the relationship of brain structure to these phenomena. Associations observed between symptoms at the time of admission to hospital and CT or MRI findings may not be detectable in a residual or deficit state. The situation may be further confounded if brain morphology is related to treatment response, or even more muddled if various symptom clusters (e.g., negative, florid psychosis, thought disorder) respond to antipsychotic medication differently in different forms of cerebral structural abnormality. Future investigations should not mix treated and untreated patients; studies are needed in which phenomenology in typical patients before and after standard treatment is assessed and related to brain structure.

Overall, despite inconsistencies in the literature, it appears that structural brain abnormality, specifically ventricular enlargement, is associated with several features of the schizophrenic deficit syndrome. Few studies provide statistically significant contradictory results. The most reproducible finding is greater cognitive dysfunction in subjects with large VBRs, followed by the relationship between greater negative symptom severity and larger ventricles. Premorbid social impairment is usually found to be associated with larger ventricles. The inverse relation between ventricular size and positive symptoms may be sensitive to treatment status, demands of the study, and whether positive symptoms are seen as a unitary phenomenon or separable into delusion-hallucination and disorganization components. Considering that ventricular enlargement is a crude and nonlocalizing measure of brain structural abnormality, and that intellectual impairment and negative symptoms apparently represent the products of complex interactions between biological vulnerabilities, medication side effects, homeostatic mechanisms, psychosocial experience and competence, and detrimental effects of institutionalization and stigma, the mere existence of such an association is remarkable.

It is hoped that the enhanced structural detail seen by MRI may identify specific sites of brain abnormality underlying the manifestations of the deficit syndrome. It can be anticipated that continued research correlating morphological alterations with physiologic, cognitive, and psychosocial aspects of schizophrenic deficit will enable researchers to advance our knowledge beyond the simplistic association between brain atrophy and "mental weakness" reported by Griesinger (1882) 108 years ago.

Chapter 10

Current View of the Type II Syndrome: Significance of Age of Onset, Intellectual Impairment, and Structural Changes in the Brain

Timothy J. Crow, M.B., F.R.C.P., Ph.D.

Chapter 10

Current View of the Type II Syndrome: Significance of Age of Onset, Intellectual Impairment, and Structural Changes in the Brain

The origin, definition, and prognostic, therapeutic, and pathogenetic significance of negative symptoms remain a matter of debate. In this chapter, I reflect on the evolution of the concept and attempt to incorporate some new findings about age of onset and asymmetries of brain structure into the debate.

In a thoughtful historical commentary, Berrios (1984) has written:

> The old distinction between positive and negative symptoms has of late been reclaimed to describe the symptomatology of schizophrenia. The commonly held view that it originated with Hughlings Jackson is grossly inaccurate.

This paper traces it back to J.H. Reynolds and shows current usage to be Reynoldian in that it does not presuppose the complex theoretical model that characterized the Jacksonian view. In particular, Berrios (1985) emphasized that the distinction has been used in the recent psychiatric literature not in the sense that positive symptoms are "release" phenomena secondary to the lesion (which in Jacksonian thinking directly induces the negative symptoms), but with the implication that positive and negative symptoms are related to independent dimensions of pathology.

An attempt by some authors to identify negative symptoms with Bleuler's class of fundamental symptoms gives the issue added significance. Bleuler (1950) regarded his category of accessory symptoms (which included delusions and hallucinations now described as positive) as secondary to the fundamental symptoms:

therefore, his position bore a formal resemblance to that of Hughlings Jackson (1889). Yet to regard "positive" symptoms as now conceived as necessarily secondary to negative symptoms is only possible if one adopts an eccentric view of negative symptoms.

Much depends, of course, on how positive and negative symptoms are to be defined. The distinction was used and developed by Wing and Brown (1970) and by Strauss et al. (1974), both of whom had contributed to the World Health Organization (1974) International Pilot Study of Schizophrenia, but it seems to have originated earlier, in the Russian literature. Thus Snezhnevsky (1968) has written that:

> Symptoms that contribute to the different schizophrenic syndromes may be pathologically productive, or so-called positive. Alternatively they may be negative symptoms, expressive of "flaws," defects, and disintegration. Both types combine as a unit, exhibiting organic interdependence and constituting the elements of a syndrome structure....However, although they form a unit, the positive and negative disturbances are not equivalent to each other. In simple schizophrenia as well as in remissions after acute attacks, negative symptoms may sometimes emerge alone without coincident positive ones. I.F. Ovchinnikov (in 1966) has pointed out that the positive and negative symptoms are disposed as if on two levels. The positive is the higher level and is characterized by marked variability....The lower or negative level by contrast is invariable....The invariability of the negative disturbances is very clearly demonstrated during contemporary therapy with modern psychotropic drugs. As a result of therapy, the positive disturbances undergo some degree of change and become more rudimentary. In some cases they may disappear altogether, and modern therapy may create a barrier to the emergence of certain features, for instance, of catatonia. The negative disturbances, however, are refractory to therapy and do not change.

Incorporated in this passage are two strands prominent in the recent literature: 1) the notion of positive and negative symptoms as independent variables with differing underlying pathology and time course, and 2) the concept that the negative symptoms are less responsive to neuroleptic medication. Some evidence from our studies at Northwick Park for the latter conclusion was one of the bases of the two-syndrome concept that I put forward a few years ago (Crow 1980a). The two-syndrome concept (see Table 10-1) was an attempt to assimilate the findings of three studies that my colleagues and I had then recently completed: 1) a computerized tomographic (CT) investigation of structural brain changes in chronic schizophrenia (Johnstone et al. 1976); 2) a study of the mechanism of the antipsychotic effect of neuroleptic drugs making use of the two stereoisomers of flupentixol (Johnstone et al. 1978b); and 3) a postmortem investigation of dopaminergic function in the basal ganglia (Owen et al. 1978).

These studies raised problems for the view that the disturbances of schizophrenia may be attributable to a single pathologic change. On the one hand, it seemed from the CT scan investigation and our studies of cognitive impairments in chronic states (Crow and Mitchell 1975; Crow and Stevens 1978) that one could envisage the disease as a slowly progressive dementing illness of early onset. On the other hand, on the basis of the flupentixol study and the postmortem investigation, much could be explained in terms of the theory formulated by Randrup and Munkvad (1965) that there is a pertubation of dopaminergic transmission that can be corrected by the receptor blockade induced by neuroleptic drugs. The two-syndrome concept suggested that there is more than one component to the underlying pathology: perhaps one can relate the more enduring negative symptoms, and the intellectual impairments with which they are

Table 10-1. The two-syndrome concept

	Type I	Type II
Characteristic symptoms	Delusions, hallucinations, thought disorder (positive symptoms)	Affective flattening, poverty of speech, loss of drive (negative symptoms)
Type of illness in which most commonly seen	Acute schizophrenia	Chronic schizophrenia, the "defect" state
Response to neuroleptic medication	Good	Poor
Outcome	Reversible	? Irreversible
Intellectual impairment	Absent	Sometimes present
Abnormal involuntary movements	Absent	Sometimes present
Postulated pathologic process	Increased dopamine receptors	Cell loss and structural change in the brain

Source. Adapted from Crow (1980a).

closely associated, to structural changes in the brain, and the more readily reversible and drug-responsive positive symptoms to a disturbance of dopaminergic transmission. This concept thus owed much to earlier discussions of the distinction between positive and negative symptoms (particularly insofar as the latter may identify a more enduring component) and attempted to relate this distinction to postulated brain changes.

DEFINITION OF NEGATIVE SYMPTOMS

It is important to note that the definition of negative symptoms that we have adopted is more restrictive than that used by many others. In our patient studies we have made use of the Krawiecka-Manchester Scale (Krawiecka et al. 1977) for rating schizophrenic symptoms. This instrument is based on a semistructured interview and allows ratings on a scale of 0 to 4. Symptoms assessed include delusions, hallucinations, and incoherence of speech, which we have taken as the group of positive symptoms (although whether incoherence of speech can always be so classified is an open question), and affective flattening and poverty of speech, which we have taken as negative symptoms. Early on, Eve Johnstone modified the scale to allow incongruity of affect to be rated separately from flattening (Silk and Tandon, Chapter 4, this volume). Experience suggests that these two symptoms often change independently and that incongruity is more closely related to the positive than to the negative group of symptoms.

Some of the problems that have arisen in defining negative symptoms are illustrated by the findings of our trial of the antipsychotic effectiveness of the two stereoisomers of flupentixol (Johnstone et al. 1978b). This study established that the alpha isomer is more effective than either the beta isomer or placebo, as predicted by the hypothesis that dopamine receptor blockade is necessary for an antipsychotic effect. We also found that the antipsychotic effect (as exemplified by the actions of alpha flupentixol) was much greater on the positive than on the negative symptoms as assessed on the Krawiecka-Manchester Scale. We concluded the negative symptoms were relatively resistant to drug treatment.

This conclusion has been challenged by Goldberg (1985), who rightly called attention to the findings of the original National Institute of Mental Health study. In this trial, he and his colleagues (Goldberg et al. 1965) had shown that drug-placebo differences were seen across a wide range of pathologic features, including some that could be described as negative in the sense that a function is diminished or lost.

In our paper, we had anticipated this discussion:

> Improvement in individual symptoms was largely confined to "positive" symptoms (Johnstone et al. 1978b). Both nonspecific and "negative" schizophrenic symptoms showed little tendency to improve or show a differential response to drug therapy.

Thus the scope of the antipsychotic effect may be more limited than was suggested by an analysis of the 1964 National Institute of Mental Health trial (Goldberg et al. 1965) in which the benefit of neuroleptic drugs appeared to be as great on some negative features of the disease (e.g., social withdrawal, lack of self-care) as on the positive symptoms. Negative symptoms (identified in a clinical interview rather than on behavior ratings as in the earlier study) are uncommon in acute schizophrenia but are prominent in the "defect state" in which neuroleptics may be less effective.

This point is borne out by the examples that Goldberg gave in his papers (1965, 1967). Among those symptoms that in various trials have been shown to respond better to neuroleptic medication than to placebo, he listed indifference to the environment, slowed speech and movements, social withdrawal, and poor self-care. Such features are undoubtedly more complex than poverty of speech and affective flattening. The distinction that Carpenter et al. (1985) made between primary and secondary negative symptoms may well be relevant. According to these authors, some negative symptoms are secondary to positive symptoms or other consequences of the disease. For example, social withdrawal may often be a response to delusions or hallucinations. Such symptoms are to be distinguished from primary negative symptoms that are enduring and resistant to treatment.

It is clear that primary negative symptoms do not exist in a vacuum but are related to other features of the disease. For example, an association with intellectual impairment was implied by the original two-syndrome concept. In the survey of 500 chronic institutionalized patients carried out by Owens and Johnstone (1980), a cluster of features (cognitive impairment, negative symptoms, behavioral disturbance, and neurologic signs) was identified that in this population was unrelated to the presence of positive symptoms. This constellation therefore can be considered to represent the features of the defect state or Type II syndrome.

Of particular interest is the presence in this constellation of neurologic signs. These include the dyskinesias that are often described as "tardive," with the implication that they are a late effect of neuroleptic administration. Such signs were seen before the introduction of such medication (Waddington and Crow 1988), however, and are present in patients who have never received such drugs (Owens et al. 1982; Rogers 1985). Thus there is doubt whether the

viewpoint that such dyskinesias are sometimes an irreversible consequence of neuroleptic administration has been properly established.
Because these movements are more closely related to the longer-term
manifestations of the disease than to its treatment, it may well be that
they should be regarded as a part of the Type II syndrome (Crow et
al. 1983).

POSSIBLE NEUROCHEMICAL CORRELATES OF THE TYPE II SYNDROME

One possible explanation of the intellectual deficits in chronic
schizophrenia is that these patients suffer from some coincidental
dementing process (e.g., senile dementia of the Alzheimer's type. An
argument against this is the fact that the incidence of cognitive
impairments in the population of patients with chronic schizophrenia
is well above the expected level in the general population (Buhrich et
al. 1988; Liddle and Crow 1984). In addition, there is no evidence
that an Alzheimer's disease process is present in the brains of these
patients. For example, in postmortem investigations, losses of
cholinergic and adrenergic neurons (as assessed by the activities of the
marker enzymes choline acetyltransferase and dopamine beta
hydroxylase, respectively) have not been detected (Crow et al. 1981).
Nor is there any compelling evidence for the presence of gliosis
(Roberts et al. 1986, 1987).

Reductions in the content of some neuropeptides, however, have
been detected by immunoassay in limbic regions and these losses are
found particularly in patients with negative symptoms. Thus losses of
cholecystokinin immunoreactivity have been detected in hippocampus and amygdala, and of somatostatin immunoreactivity in hippocampus (Ferrier et al. 1983b; Roberts et al. 1983). Apart from a
reduction of cholecystokinin in temporal cortex, changes in these
peptides in other areas were not observed, and no alterations were
seen in the content of other neuropeptides (e.g., substance P,
neurotensin, and vasoactive intestinal peptide) in a number of brain
areas. A possible explanation for these findings is that in patients with
the Type II syndrome, there is a loss of the small interneurons
containing the peptides cholecystokinin and somatostatin in hippocampus and amygdala. Of further interest is the observation that
cholecystokinin-binding sites are reduced in the hippocampus, temporal cortex, and an area of frontal cortex (Farmery et al. 1985),
although these losses have not been related to a specific clinical
picture.

Two forms of the enzyme monoamine oxidase are present in the
brain. The A form, for which phenylethylamine is a substrate, is

located mainly in neurons. The B form, for which benzylamine is a substrate, is found preferentially in glia. In a postmortem investigation in schizophrenic patients (Owen et al. 1987), the activity of the A form was unchanged but significant reductions in activity of the type B enzyme were observed in areas of frontal and temporal cortex and amygdala. These reductions were seen particularly in patients with affective flattening and poverty of speech. Because of the location of the B form of the enzyme, these changes seem unlikely to be related to transmitter function but may indicate some alteration in glial function or number.

THE MEANING OF THE STRUCTURAL CHANGES IN THE BRAIN

Following the early CT scan studies from Northwick Park (Johnstone et al. 1976) and St. Elizabeths Hospital (Weinberger et al. 1979), a large number of investigations of patients with schizophrenia have been conducted. There is a degree of consensus (e.g., Stahl et al. 1988) that when patients with the more chronic forms of the disease are included, mean ventricular size is modestly increased. It is also clear that this enlargement cannot be attributed to past physical treatments (Owens et al. 1985).

There is less agreement concerning clinical correlates. Although there is a general trend toward finding ventricular size to be related to behavioral deterioration and the more chronic forms of the disease, significant associations with individual features of the defect state are not always found (Crow and Johnstone 1986). Thus correlations with affective flattening and other negative symptoms, and with intellectual impairment, are found in some studies but not in others. In our own investigation of more than 100 patients with chronic schizophrenia (Owens et al. 1985), lateral ventricular size was significantly related to behavioral deterioration and the presence of dyskinesias, but not to negative symptoms or intellectual impairment. Although such correlations have been reported in some other studies (e.g., Kemali et al. 1987; Kling et al. 1983; Takahashi et al. 1982; Williams et al. 1985), the absence of a consistent relationship is puzzling.

Some insight may be provided by an examination of age of onset as a predictor of outcome and the relationship between brain structure and other clinical features (Johnstone et al. 1989). In a population of chronic patients, we found that when other relevant variables (e.g., age and duration of illness) were controlled, age of onset predicted a number of aspects of outcome. Thus patients who were first admitted to the hospital at an age below the mode for the group as a whole (25 years for males and 28 years for females) were more likely than those who were first admitted at a later age to show negative symptoms, intellectual impairment (e.g., age disorientation), and behavioral deterioration. Moreover, some associations between structural change and cognitive function were seen in the early onset group that were absent in the total sample. These correlations were with brain area (which was significantly reduced in these patients by comparison with age-matched psychiatric controls) rather than with enlargement of the third or lateral ventricles.

The findings indicate that age of onset is a determinant of the relationship between the structure of the brain and the cognitive impairments that are one consequence of the schizophrenic disease process. They suggest that these associations are established early in the course of the illness. They are compatible with the notion that the disease itself is an anomaly of development rather than a degenerative process attributable to an exogenous pathogen.

On this basis, it might be expected that age of onset would be a determinant of the structural changes in schizophrenia. Surprisingly, we found that the three measures (lateral and third ventricular area and brain area) that distinguished patients with schizophrenia from other subjects did not separate patients with early age of onset from those with late age of onset. A further structural index—the difference between the widths of the two sides of the brain in the posterior segments—did distinguish these groups, however. Patients with early age of onset had significant ($P < .01$) reductions in the relative width of the left hemisphere in measures taken in the occipital and temporal regions (Crow et al. 1989b). It seemed from these findings as though early onset of a schizophrenic illness might arrest the development of the normal asymmetries present in the posterior part of the brain.

This finding may be a clue to the meaning of the structural changes in the brain, suggesting the possibility that the core disturbance involves the mechanisms controlling the development of asymmetry in the human brain. Some other findings suggest that the structural changes in the brain in schizophrenia are lateralized. Thus, using air encephalographic comparisons of acute and chronic patients with schizophrenia, Haug (1982) found that the latter had larger temporal horns and that the differences were greater on the left side. In their CT study of monozygotic twins discordant for schizophrenia, Reveley et al. (1987) found a reduction in CT scan density in the affected twin on the left side of the brain in comparison with the unaffected twin. Such a reduction was not present in nonschizophrenic twin controls. Presumably it reflects an enlargement in cerebrospinal fluid spaces that does not appear on the CT image. In a postmortem study, we (Brown et al. 1986) found that width of the parahippocampal gyrus was smaller in schizophrenic patients than in affective patients; this difference again was significantly greater in the left hemisphere. In a further study (Crow et al. 1989b), we assessed radiologically the area of the various components of the lateral ventricle after introduction of radio-opaque medium; enlargement was relatively selective to the temporal horn and highly ($P < .001$) selective to the left hemisphere. Although temporal horn enlargement was seen in Alzheimer-type dementia, this enlargement showed no predilection for the left side of the brain.

The asymmetries in the human brain are localized in the temporal lobe and include particularly the planum temporale (Geschwind and Levitsky 1968). They may relate to handedness, which itself could be determined by a simple Mendelian gene (Annett 1985). Thus this gene may be the focus of the disturbance in schizophrenia (Crow 1984, 1989a).

CONCLUSIONS

A constellation of features that occurs in chronic schizophrenia may define the Type II syndrome or defect state. This syndrome is relatively nonresponsive to neuroleptic medication and is closely related to the chronic impairments of schizophrenia. These features include 1) negative symptoms (e.g., affective flattening and poverty of speech) relatively restrictively defined (i.e., so as to exclude features that may be secondary to positive symptoms); 2) intellectual impairments, which may be severe; 3) behavioral deterioration; and 4) dyskinesias. The clinical correlates of structural change in the brain have varied from one study to another, but when present tend to have been among the features of the Type II syndrome. Some evidence from postmortem investigations suggests that the Type II syndrome is associated with losses of cholecystokinin neurons in limbic regions and a reduction of type B monoamine oxidase (which may be located in glial cells).

Age of onset is an important determinant of the features of the defect state; patients with an early onset are more likely to develop negative symptoms and intellectual impairments than those whose onset of illness is later. Age of onset also may influence the relationship between brain structure and cognitive function. Such findings promote a developmental view of schizophrenia in suggesting that the disease may be associated with an anomaly of brain growth. According to some radiologic and postmortem findings, the focus of the structural change may be in the mechanisms that determine the development of asymmetries in the human brain.

Chapter 11

A Developmental Model of Negative Syndromes in Schizophrenia

Sukdeb Mukherjee, M.D.
Ravinder Reddy, M.D.
David B. Schnur, M.D.

Chapter 11

A Developmental Model of Negative Syndromes in Schizophrenia

Negative symptoms are commonly regarded as behavioral manifestations of a deficit state—the diminution of expected normal functions. Such impairments, particularly in schizophrenic patients, occur in multiple functional dimensions. Which of the myriad behavioral deficits should be regarded as negative symptoms remains controversial. For example, Andreasen (1985) included five dimensions of functioning under negative symptoms: affective flattening, alogia, avolition-apathy, anhedonia-asociality, and attentional impairment. By contrast, Crow (1985) proposed a narrower definition that incorporated only affective flattening and poverty of speech. Carpenter et al. (1988) emphasized the distinction between primary and secondary negative symptoms and suggested that enduring negative symptoms better represent the deficit state. These are not mere academic issues; the significance of "negative symptoms" is ultimately determined by its component items.

Regardless of issues of definition, negative symptoms are not invariant with regard to their time of appearance or stability during the course of illness. The recognition that they may appear insidiously and antedate the onset of florid psychosis has led to speculation that premorbid social dysfunction may be an antecedent to the subsequent development of negative symptoms (Andreasen 1985; Crow 1980a; Strauss et al. 1977; Zubin 1985). This idea is intriguing in light of evidence that early pathologic influences, such as exposure to a viral

This work was supported in part by NIMH grant MH-41961, a grant from the Van Ameringen Foundation, and the New York State Office of Mental Health. We thank the staff, past and present, of the Special Treatment Unit at Creedmoor for their assistance in the care of the patients and data collection.

epidemic during the second trimester of gestation or perinatal complications, may be relevant to the pathogenesis of schizophrenia (McNeil and Kaij 1978; Mednick et al. 1988). Moreover, neuropathologic findings consistent with an early developmental pathology have been found in postmortem brain studies of patients diagnosed as suffering from schizophrenia during their lifetime (e.g., Jakob and Beckmann 1986). Various hypotheses implicating brain developmental and maturational processes in the pathogenesis of schizophrenia have been proposed (Conrad and Scheibel 1987; Crow 1984; Feinberg 1983; Weinberger 1987). Thus it may be meaningful to examine the negative symptoms of schizophrenia from a developmental perspective. The basic principles of this approach have been discussed by Rutter (1988).

Impairments in a variety of functional dimensions are known to occur long before the onset of florid psychosis in schizophrenic patients (Fish 1977; Parnas et al. 1986; Strauss et al. 1977). Although the emphasis on psychosis as a hallmark of schizophrenia has led to conceptualizing such early impairments as premorbid, it remains to be determined whether they are indeed premorbid or early manifestations of the disease process. It is imperative to determine whether such impairment of function reflects a deterioration from a prior better level of functioning or an initial failure to develop a normal repertoire of functioning. If the former, the period of life when this deterioration occurs needs to be considered. It is generally assumed that functional deterioration in schizophrenic patients occurs subsequent to the onset of psychosis (Bleuler 1983; Ciompi 1983). This view stems from the failure to recognize that premorbid functioning is a dynamic and evolving process, and that deterioration in functioning can occur prior to the onset of manifest psychosis. Furthermore, although Strauss et al. (1977) earlier cautioned against considering premorbid adjustment as being absolute, temporally invariant, and unrelated to the subject's age, premorbid deterioration of functioning has not been considered in previous research. A history of poor premorbid functioning has been reported to be associated with prominent negative symptoms after the onset of illness (Andreasen and Olsen 1982; Kay and Opler 1987; Keefe et al. 1989; Kolakowska et al. 1985; Opler et al. 1984). These studies, however, did not address premorbid functioning during childhood. Thus it cannot be determined whether the premorbid impairment during adolescence observed in these studies reflects continuity of poor function from childhood onward, or deterioration from previous better levels of function.

Premorbid impairment may occur in different functional dimensions, and these dimensions may need to be examined separately. The studies mentioned above, for example, used global measures of broadly defined negative symptoms and did not examine separately the relations of premorbid adjustment to discrete dimensions of negative symptoms. The presence of prominent negative symptoms has been associated with fewer years of formal education and poor performance on tests of cognitive and mental functions (Andreasen and Olsen 1982; Johnstone et al. 1978a; Kay and Opler 1987). There is evidence that poor premorbid intellectual functioning is associated with a greater likelihood of subsequent development of schizophrenia (Aylward et al. 1984; Watt et al. 1984). Negative symptoms have been linked with neuropsychological performance deficits that suggest early developmental compromise of cognitive functions (Bilder et al. 1985; Kay and Opler 1987). This relationship, however, may not hold true across all negative symptoms. Using the Scale for the Assessment of Negative Symptoms (SANS) (Andreasen 1983), we found neuro-psychological impairments of language and memory functions to be associated with global alogia and attentional impairment, but not with affective flattening, avolition-apathy, or anhedonia-asociality (Bilder et al. 1985). Thus various negative symptom dimensions may have differential relations to developmental events.

The primary aim of this preliminary report is to examine the relationship between selected aspects of premorbid functioning and negative symptoms in schizophrenic patients. Specifically, the relations of negative symptoms to childhood premorbid functioning and premorbid deterioration of functioning at the transition from childhood to early adolescence are reviewed.

SUBJECTS AND METHODS

The sample consisted of 40 (25 men) schizophrenic patients admitted at the New York State Psychiatric Institute affiliated research unit at Creedmoor Psychiatric Center. Those with mental retardation, alcohol and drug dependence, serious medical conditions requiring treatment, and a history of head injury were excluded. Inclusion was limited to patients who were 45 years old or younger to minimize possible effects of aging on major dependent measures. A DSM-III (American Psychiatric Association 1980) diagnosis of schizophrenic disorder was established on the basis of independent interviews by two research psychiatrists. The patients had a mean (±SD) age of 31.1 5.1 years (range, 20–43) and a mean of 11.9 ± 2.1 years of formal education. The mean age at onset of illness was 19.5 ± 5.0 years (range, 14–35), and the mean duration of illness was 11.5 ± 5.5 years (range, 5–20). No patient was in an acute state of psychosis at the time of assessment.

Premorbid functioning was assessed using the Premorbid Adjustment Scale (PAS) (Cannon-Spoor et al. 1982), in which functioning is assessed separately for childhood, early adolescence, late adolescence, and adulthood. PAS ratings were made by a research psychiatrist, who usually was also the primary treating physician at the research unit. Sources of information included extensive interviews with patients and family members, school reports when available, hospital records, and reports from previous treatment facilities. Only items pertaining to childhood (through age 11 years) and early adolescence (ages 12–15 years) were considered in this study. The childhood subscale of the PAS consists of four items: social accessibility-withdrawal, peer relationships, scholastic performance, and adaptation to school. The early adolescence subscale contains, in addition, an item assessing sociosexual functioning. The item scores of social accessibility-withdrawal and peer relationship were summed and then divided by the highest possible score to provide a social functioning score that ranged from 0 to 1, with higher scores indicating poorer functioning. Scholastic performance and adaptation to school were similarly combined to derive a separate school performance score. Calculations were made separately for each age period. A premorbid index of change was computed for each composite measure (social functioning and school performance) by subtracting the childhood score from the corresponding early adolescence score. Thus positive scores indicated deterioration and negative scores improvement in functioning from childhood to early adolescence. Sociosexual functioning, which is not rated for the childhood period, was examined as a separate item.

Negative symptoms were assessed during baseline evaluations using the SANS, which comprises five global subscales (affective flattening, alogia, avolition-apathy, anhedonia, and attentional impairment), including a variable number of items that are rated on a severity scale of 0 to 5. In an earlier investigation of 18 patients, we found that SANS global measures remained stable over a 1- to 3-year follow-up period (Schnur, unpublished data). The measure of global affective flattening was modified and a mean score was computed after excluding the items of inappropriate affect and subjective experience of emotions. Only the modified measure of affective flattening was used in this study.

Premorbid functioning scores and negative symptoms were initially examined as continuous measures, and two-tailed values were used for all tests of significance.

RESULTS

Distributions of the various PAS scores did not show significant departures from normality. Specifically, none of the measures had a bimodal distribution. Males consistently had higher scores (poorer functioning) than females, but a statistically significant difference was found only for early adolescent school performance ($t = 2.2, P < .05$) and sociosexual functioning ($t = 3.2, P < .01$). None of the SANS global scores of negative symptoms was correlated with age, sex, or years of formal education. Age at onset of illness was significantly and inversely correlated only with alogia ($r = -.33, P < .05$) and avolition-apathy ($r = -.36, P < .05$). Duration of illness was significantly correlated with alogia ($r = .42, P < .01$), avolition-apathy ($r = .50, P < .01$), anhedonia-asociality ($r = .43, P < .01$), and attentional impairment ($r = .37, P < .05$), but not with affective flattening ($r = .25$).

Premorbid Functioning and Negative Symptoms

Neither social functioning nor school performance during childhood was correlated with any of the five SANS global subscale scores. Affective blunting, but no other global subscale score of the SANS, was significantly correlated with early adolescent social functioning ($r = .40, P < .02$) and sociosexual functioning ($r = .48, P < .01$). Since our earlier work had suggested that alogia and attentional impairment may reflect developmental compromise of cognitive functions (Bilder et al. 1985), the failure to observe a relationship between these negative symptoms and premorbid school performance was somewhat surprising. When the alogia items of poverty of speech and poverty of content of speech were examined separately, it became obvious that these items had differential relations to premorbid functioning that were obscured when the global alogia score was examined (Table 11-1). Poverty of content of speech was significantly associated with poorer school performance during both childhood ($r = .34, P = .04$) and early adolescence ($r = .32, P = .05$). On the other hand, poverty of speech was significantly correlated with school performance during early adolescence ($r = .35, P = .03$), but not during childhood. Thus poverty of content of speech appears to be related to impaired school performance from childhood onward. By contrast, poverty of speech appeared to reflect a process involving premorbid functional deterioration. When patients were categorized into good and poor childhood school performance groups based on published means (0.20) for these items of the PAS in normal subjects, the mean ($\pm$SD) attentional impairment rating was significantly higher in the 14 patients with poor childhood school performance (3.2 ± 1.6) than in the 26 patients with good childhood school performance (1.8 ± 1.6) ($t = 2.4, P = .02$). Mean poverty of content of speech rating was also significantly higher in those with poor childhood school performance (2.9 ± 1.4) than in those with good childhood school performance (1.2 ± 1.3) (t = 3.6, P < .001). Categorization did not yield a significant association between poor school performance and affective blunting, poverty of speech, anhedonia-asociality, or avolition-apathy. Negative symptoms scores did not differ between the 24 patients with good social functioning and the 16 patients with poor social functioning during childhood. Thus only attentional impairment and poverty of content of speech were found to be associated with childhood dysfunction, specifically involving school performance.

Premorbid Deterioration and Negative Symptoms

On the average, school performance showed significant deterioration from childhood to early adolescence (P < .001); social functioning showed a more modest deterioration (P < .10). Deterioration of social functioning, however, was more marked when childhood and late adolescence scores were compared (P < .001). No significant association was observed between the measures of premorbid deterioration and age, sex, age at onset of illness, duration of illness, or years of formal education.

As shown in Table 11-1, premorbid deterioration of social functioning from childhood to early adolescence was significantly correlated with global affective blunting and poverty of speech, but not with poverty of content of speech or global scores of alogia, anhedonia-asociality, avolition-apathy, or attentional impairment. Premorbid social deterioration was significantly correlated with early

Table 11-1. Correlations between measures of premorbid functioning and negative symptoms

SANS measures of negative symptoms	Childhood school performance	Premorbid social deterioration
Global affective	.08	.34*
Global affective flattening	.22	.26
Poverty of speech	.13	.35*
Poverty of content of speech	.34*	.02
Global avolition-apathy	.21	.12
Global anhedonia-asociality	.24	.23
Global attentional impairment	.21	.01

Note. None of the negative symptoms were correlated with either childhood social functioning or premorbid deterioration of school performance. SANS = Scale for the Assessment of Negative Symptoms.
*P < .05.

adolescent sociosexual functioning ($r = .40$, $P < .01$), which earlier was found to be associated with affective blunting. By contrast, premorbid deterioration of school performance was not related to any dimension of negative symptoms.

COMMENTS

The findings of this study suggest that, from a developmental perspective, there are at least two discrete dimensions of negative symptoms. One dimension is characterized by affective blunting and poverty of speech and appears to be related to deterioration of social functioning at puberty. The second dimension is characterized by attentional impairment and poverty of content of speech and appears to reflect an early developmental compromise of cognitive functions and poor school performance. The negative symptoms of anhedonia-asociality and avolition-apathy do not appear to be specifically linked to either developmental stage.

Premorbid deterioration has not been examined previously. The PAS offers a unique opportunity to examine functional deterioration at a specific life period: puberty, the transition from childhood to early adolescence. We propose that deterioration of functioning around puberty reflects a specific pathologic process. In our study, deterioration was noted at this time to occur both in school performance and in social functioning, yet affective blunting and poverty of speech was selectively related to the latter. In a separate study, we found cortical sulcal prominence on computed tomography scans to be related to deterioration of school performance, but not to social functioning (Mukherjee et al., unpublished data). Cortical sulcal prominence is not associated with negative symptoms in our patients. Since some patients showed deterioration in both dimensions of functioning, these processes are not mutually exclusive. More likely, a common pathologic process underlies these changes and expresses itself variably in discrete secondary processes. The consequences of premorbid deterioration are then determined by the dimension of functioning involved. One of these consequences may be manifest in deterioration of school performance and increased sulcal prominence, another in deterioration of social functioning and in negative symptoms such as affective flattening and poverty of speech. There may be other consequences of premorbid deterioration of function that remain to be elucidated. Confirmation that a pathologic process occurs around puberty requires, at minimum, demonstration of temporal specificity for the observed correlations. We therefore examined the relationship of affective blunting and poverty of speech to deterioration in social functioning from early adolescence to late adolescence. This later premorbid deterioration was not significantly correlated with either affective flattening or poverty of speech. Further, these negative symptoms were not related to childhood functional impairments. We have also examined other indicators of early developmental insult, such as estimated premorbid intellectual functioning, birth weight, and pregnancy and birth complications. None of these indicators was associated with affective flattening or poverty of speech in our patients (unpublished data). Thus affective flattening and poverty of speech appear to be related to a pathologic process occurring specifically around puberty. The nature of this putative process remains to be determined. Consideration of normal brain maturational events that occur around puberty, however, may suggest possible avenues for exploration in future research.

The nervous system appears to be genetically programmed to produce an excessive number of neurons and synapses and to seek an optimal quantitative balance through processes of neuronal death and synapse elimination as part of normal maturation (Purves and Lichtman 1985). This initial overproduction of neurons and their synaptic contacts may confer a biological advantage by reducing the genetic load that would otherwise be required to program selectively the enormous number of synapses in the brain. Neuronal death occurs early in development and is believed to be completed in humans by 2 years of age. In contrast, synapse elimination may be a more protracted process. In a postmortem study of normal human brains, Huttenlocher (1979) found that synaptic density increased to an apparent maximum by the age of 2 to 3 years and then declined steeply to adult levels in late childhood and early adolescence. He concluded that synapse elimination occurs as a late developmental event in the human cerebral cortex. A temporal pattern of change as a function of development virtually identical to that noted by Huttenlocher for synaptic density has been observed for delta sleep time and delta wave amplitude (Feinberg 1983), local cerebral metabolic rate for glucose (LCMRGlc) using positron emission tomography (Chugani et al. 1987), and pineal melatonin levels (Hartmann et al. 1982; Waldhauser et al. 1984).

Feinberg (1983) earlier proposed that faulty synapse elimination may be involved in the pathology of schizophrenia. If indeed the developmental changes in slow-wave sleep, LCMRGlc, and pineal melatonin functions during development reflect brain maturational changes related to synapse elimination, deviations from expected normal patterns in these physiologic functions should be noted in schizophrenic patients with negative symptoms. Such associations between negative symptoms and abnormalities in slow-wave sleep

(Ganguli et al. 1987; Tandon et al. 1989a; van Kammen et al. 1988), nocturnal melatonin levels (Ferrier et al. 1982), and increased LCMRGlc (Szechtman et al. 1988) have in fact been reported in schizophrenic patients. Whether these physiologic abnormalities are related to deterioration of functioning at the transition from childhood to adolescence remains to be examined. The peak period of synapse elimination and the above physiologic changes (the transition from childhood to adolescence), however, corresponds to the period at which we found premorbid deterioration of functioning to occur. Although temporal correspondence clearly is not a sufficient basis for establishing a causal relation, it does suggest that such a possibility be considered.

The mechanisms regulating normal synapse elimination are not yet fully understood. It appears that genetic as well as experiential influences are critical to this process (Haracz 1985; Purves and Lichtman 1985). Rakic et al. (1986) suggested that if experience alters synaptic number during development, it does so by influencing the selective survival of certain synapses and not by regulating their initial formation. It is conceivable that, in addition to possible genetic misprogramming, interactions between specific abnormalities of attentional and information-processing functions and adverse experiences during early life may contribute to pathologic maturation and thus to premorbid deterioration, affective flattening, and poverty of speech in schizophrenic patients. The particular appeal of this hypothesis is that, in invoking a neurobiologic model, it leaves open the possibility that experiential factors also may contribute to the development of negative symptoms.

The second dimension of negative symptoms consists of attentional impairment and poverty of content of speech and appears to be related to an early developmental pathology. These "cognitive" negative symptoms were associated with poor school performance from childhood onward, but not with premorbid social functioning. This observation is consonant with our earlier finding that impaired neuropsychological performance is associated with attentional impairment and alogia, suggesting a long-standing, static dysfunction: a pattern consistent with early developmental compromise (Bilder et al. 1985). Further, we have found that both poor estimated premorbid intellectual ability and a lower current verbal IQ were associated with attentional impairment and poverty of content of speech, but not with affective blunting and poverty of speech (unpublished data). Whether the hypotheses implicating early developmental pathology in schizophrenia (e.g., Conrad and Scheibel 1987; Crow in Chapter 10 of this volume; Mednick et al. 1988) might account for the observed relationships remains to be examined in future research.

We were unable to account for the symptom complexes of avolition-apathy and anhedonia-asociality within a developmental model. Both symptoms were unrelated to the premorbid measures examined but significantly associated with a longer duration of illness, suggesting that these symptoms may be functions of the chronicity of the illness. Another possibility is that developmental variables not examined in this study account for these symptoms. Recent findings from the Danish High Risk Study, for example, indicate that failure to show an autonomic orienting response to innocuous stimuli during the premorbid period is associated at follow-up with greater avolition-apathy, but not affective flattening or alogia (Cannon et al. 1990).

Our findings have major implications for the definition of negative symptoms. Within a developmental perspective, negative symptoms do not appear to represent a unitary syndrome. By contrast, a narrower definition of negative symptoms limited to affective flattening and poverty of speech may be more homogenous. Although the general concept of negative symptoms has been of considerable heuristic value and has succeeded in generating research findings and hypotheses, the time may have arrived for abandoning this general construct and examining separately its discrete components. As shown in this study, this approach may yield findings that have potential significance for an understanding of etiologic and developmental aspects of schizophrenia. Findings from our work would have generated different conclusions if we had examined only global measures of negative symptom and premorbid functioning.

That there may be more than one pathologic process in schizophrenia, each with its independent antecedents and consequences, has been proposed (Crow 1980b; Strauss et al. 1974, 1977). Our preliminary findings suggest that negative symptoms may involve multiple processes. Such speculation does not necessarily mean that there are discrete etiologies of schizophrenia or categorical subtypes of patients. The different pathologic dimensions are not mutually exclusive and are often seen in the same patient. It is likely that a unitary primary pathogenic event occurs early during development, possibly in utero, and interactions between this event and "protective" or other modifying factors result variably in different secondary pathologic processes that ultimately manifest themselves in the signs and symptoms on which we base our diagnoses. Thus the heterogeneity of clinical and biological features of schizophrenia may signify variable representations of different secondary pathologic processes rather than discrete subtypes of the disorder. An implication of this view is that the signs and symptoms by which we presently characterize schizophrenia may represent secondary complications of a more fundamental pathology that may not be revealed through a purely phenomenological approach.

Chapter 12

Genetic and Environmental Correlates of the Positive and Negative Syndromes

Alice Foerster, M.B., M.R.C.P.
Shon W. Lewis, M.B., M.R.C.P.
Robin M. Murray, M.B., F.R.C.P.

Chapter 12

Genetic and Environmental Correlates of the Positive and Negative Syndromes

Even as historical arguments have raged concerning the boundaries of schizophrenia and its relation to other psychiatric conditions, many and varied attempts have been made to subtype schizophrenia by symptoms, often in the hope of finding etiologically homogenous groups. In consequence, the four classic Kraepelinian subtypes have been supplemented by dichotimizing classifications, including the paranoid versus nonparanoid distinction of Tsuang and Winokur (1974), the H versus P subtypes of Farmer et al. (1983), the Type I versus Type II (Crow 1980a), and the negative versus positive divisions (Andreasen and Olsen 1982; Wing and Brown 1978) that are the subject of this volume. Some of these classifications have been derived empirically by multivariate statistical studies of patient groups (e.g., Farmer et al. 1983). Others, such as that of Crow, have arisen out of a more theoretical approach. In fact, the empirical and theoretically derived systems have more in common than one might expect (Table 12-1). Schizophrenic illnesses with positive symptoms tend to be labeled as paranoid if they are chronic, or schizoaffective if they remit; those with negative symptoms tend to be classified as nonparanoid or process.

Those seeking to establish different etiologies for the positive and negative subtypes have struggled with the degree to which the subtypes are truly different. Whatever definition of negative and positive characteristics researchers have employed, they have found overlap cross-sectionally, but even more so longitudinally. Crow (1985) stated firmly that Type I and Type II do not represent different types of schizophrenic illness and acknowledged that overlapping

Supported by grants from the Medical Research Council and Mental Health Foundation.

Table 12-1. Schizophrenic subtypes

Author	Subtypes	Characteristics
Tsuang and Winokur (1974)	Paranoid	Well-organized delusions or hallucinations; affective behavioral symptoms and disorganized thoughts not prominent; later age of onset (after 25); married or employed; no family history of schizophrenia
	Nonparanoid	Inappropriate or flat affect, bizarre behavior, disorganized thoughts; organized delusions or hallucinations not prominent; early age of onset (before 25); unmarried or unemployed; family history of schizophrenia
Farmer et al. (1983)	P type	Well-organized delusions; later onset; good premorbid adjustment
	H type	Bizarre behavior, incoherent speech, blunted affect; early onset; poor premorbid adjustment; family history of schizophrenia
Crow (1980a)	Type I	Prominent delusions, hallucinations and thought disorder; acute onset; good response to medication; no intellectual impairment; good recovery; increased dopamine receptors
	Type II	Affective flattening; poverty of speech; loss of drive, insidious onset; poor response to medication; sometimes intellectual impairment; poor recovery; cell loss and structural changes in the brain

Andreasen and Olsen (1982)	Positive	Prominent delusions, hallucinations; formal thought disorder and bizarre behavior; good premorbid adjustment; less evidence of cognitive dysfunction; nonchronic course; less evidence of increased ventricle-brain ratio
	Mixed	Neither negative nor positive symptoms prominent
	Negative	Prominent affective flattening, alogia, avolition, anhedonia, and attentional impairment; poor premorbid adjustment; evidence of cognitive dysfunction; chronic course; more evidence of increased ventricle-brain ratio
Liddle (1987a)	Reality distortion	Delusions of reference, bizarre delusions, auditory hallucinations
	Disorganization	Formal thought disorder, inappropriate affect, poor self-care
	Psychomotor poverty	Poverty of speech and movement, blunted affect, anergia

positive and negative features are common, particularly in chronic patients. Symptom overlap with depression is also frequent (Andreasen and Olsen 1982; Pogue-Geile and Harrow 1984; Kay et al. 1986b, 1986c). Furthermore, several groups have found correlations between the severity of positive symptoms in the acute phase and of negative symptoms in the post-acute phase of schizophrenia (Kay et al. 1986c; Pogue-Geile and Harrow 1984, 1987b).

In an effort to clarify the situation, Liddle (1987a) examined 40 patients with chronic positive and negative symptoms and reported that factor analysis identified three overlapping syndromes. One syndrome, the "reality distortion" syndrome, was equivalent to a positive symptom group. A second, the "psychomotor poverty group," was similar to the previously postulated negative symptom group. The third, "disorganized" syndrome, was characterized by formal thought disorder and had been variously assigned by other authors to positive or negative groups. These findings, which subsequently have been replicated in a second sample of 57 chronic schizophrenic patients (Liddle et al. 1989), bear out the findings of Bilder et al. (1985). The latter study also found three syndromes on factor analysis: one characterized by delusions and hallucinations, one by poverty of speech and blunted affect, and a third by formal thought disorder. Taken together, these studies offer impressive support for the validity of the positive-negative distinction, along with a third largely unrelated dimension of thought disorder.

There have been many attempts to find features associated with negative symptoms. The most frequently reported associations, although not universally confirmed, appear to be poor premorbid adjustment and educational achievement (Andreasen and Olsen 1982; Opler et al. 1984; Johnstone et al. 1981; Pogue-Geile and Harrow 1984, 1987a), cognitive impairment (Johnstone et al. 1978a, 1981; Liddle 1987b), and poor outcome (Biehl et al. 1986; Pogue-Geile and Harrow 1985, 1987b). The relationship between structural brain abnormalities and negative symptoms appears more complex than originally envisaged, and although it was not part of his initial definition, Crow (1985) has now added involuntary movements to the Type II syndrome.

GENETIC FACTORS

There is convincing evidence that genetic factors play an important etiologic role in schizophrenia (Gottesman and Shields 1982; Murray et al. 1986), but no straightforward pattern of transmission has been identified. Multifactorial polygenic inheritance, a single major locus, and a major gene against a polygenic background have all been suggested to explain the data (McGue et al. 1985; McGuffin et al. 1987; O'Rourke et al. 1982). It seems most likely that schizophrenia is a multifactorial disease, involving several genes as well as environmental factors, but that does not mean that it is multifactorial in each case. There probably will be cases, such as those from multiply affected families, where the disease shows a dominant inheritance pattern with high penetrance, but other cases will exist that are wholly attributable to environmental causes (phenocopies). Then there will be the majority, in which the etiology involves a combination of genetic predisposition and environmental factors.

Is there any evidence that genetic factors are more important in the pathogenesis of positive, as opposed to negative, schizophrenia? Kay et al. (1986c) reported that the occurrence of negative symptoms was correlated positively with a family history of major psychiatric disorder but negatively with a family history of affective disorder. Few details were given, however, and no satisfactory studies have estimated morbid risk in the relatives of positive versus negative probands. Therefore, we must seek indirect evidence.

Scharfetter (1981) examined relatives of index cases with the classic Kraepelinian subtypes of schizophrenia. Although the different subtypes were not totally genetically distinct, there was some tendency toward a similar picture being found in probands and their relatives. The increased risk for relatives of catatonic or hebephrenic over paranoid cases found in this study is now well replicated. In a review of nine studies, Kendler and Davis (1981) found the risk for first-degree relatives of paranoid schizophrenic patients to be between 0.7% and 11.1%, and for those of hebephrenic schizophrenic patients to be between 1.8% and 18%. Thus the paranoid subtype appears to be less familial than the hebephrenic. This observation does not, however, prove that the two types are etiologically discrete. For example, the data also fit a two-threshold multifactorial model in which hebephrenia lies at the more extreme end of a continuum of polygenic liability than paranoia. Such a continuum of liability would explain the greater severity and familiality of hebephrenia, as well as its earlier onset (McGuffin et al. 1987).

Kendler et al. (1985) showed that when schizophrenia is broadly defined, the relatives of schizophrenic patients have a relative risk of 9 compared to relatives of surgical controls; when schizophrenia is defined by DSM-III (American Psychiatric Association 1980) criteria, the absolute risk declines, but the relative risk rises to 18. DSM-III criteria rely not only on phenomenology, but also on evidence of prolonged impairment and poor social functioning, characteristics related to the negative syndrome. The fact that the use of these criteria increases familiality suggests that the same might be found for negative symptoms.

The Maudsley schizophrenic twin sample of Gottesman and Shields (1972) has also been reexamined to establish which diagnostic criteria appear to be most heritable. These studies (Farmer et al. 1987; McGuffin et al. 1984) have shown that the DSM-III criteria, Feighner's criteria (Feighner et al. 1972), and Research Diagnostic Criteria (Spitzer et al. 1978) are all highly heritable, but that Schneider's first-rank symptoms (Schneider 1959) define a type of schizophrenia that does not appear at all "genetic." Since the first two of these criteria contain some elements of the negative syndrome, whereas Schneiderian criteria rely heavily on positive symptoms, this relative heritability could be taken as indirect evidence for the greater importance of genetic factors in the negative versus positive syndrome. Operationalized criteria for Crow's Type I, Type II, and mixed types were applied to the same sample (McGuffin et al. 1987). Monozygotic concordance was highest as compared to dizygotic concordance for the mixed type (Table 12-2): the difference in concordance was smaller for a pure Type I syndrome. Unfortunately, too few patients met the pure Type II criteria to allow firm conclusions to be drawn.

Another group (Dworkin et al. 1984) reanalyzed data from five previously published twin studies, retrospectively applying ratings of negative and positive symptoms to summaries of 151 monozygotic

Table 12-2. Probandwise monozygotic and dizygotic concordance by subtypes

Subtypes		Monozygotic concordance (%)	Dizygotic concordance (%)
Tsuang and Winokur (1974)		40	7
	Paranoid		
	Nonparanoid	62	15
Farmer et al. (1983)		33	6
	P type		
	H type	79	18
Crow (1980)		53	19
	Type I		
	Mixed type	64	0
	Type II	0	0

Source. Adapted from McGuffin et al. (1987).

twin pairs. Dividing probands into those with "high" and "low" negative symptoms, they found higher concordance rates among the former. A parallel analysis was made for positive symptoms, but no relationship was found. The authors concluded that negative symptoms may be characteristic of that type of schizophrenia in which there is a greater genetic component.

A subsequent analysis (Dworkin et al. 1988) showed that probands from the concordant pairs not only had more negative symptoms, but also poorer premorbid adjustment, fewer paranoid symptoms, and earlier ages of onset than probands from discordant pairs (i.e., several of the features of the negative syndrome). Unfortunately, one must point out the methodological deficiencies in this study. These include the use of twin summaries not prepared for this purpose, the pooling of data of very different quality, and the lack of blindness in much of the data collected. The first and third of these criticisms also apply to the reanalyses of the Maudsley sample.

Other studies suggest that genetic factors may also be important in protecting against the development of negative symptoms. Several carefully executed controlled family studies have found an increased prevalence of unipolar, but not bipolar, affective disorder in the relatives of schizophrenic probands, the most recent being Gershon et al. (1988). In a review of the literature, Kendler and Tsuang (1988) concluded that a family history of affective disorder conferred a better prognosis on schizophrenia, a hypothesis that they confirmed in their own sample. Recent biological research supports the idea that schizophrenia with a family history of affective disorder is separate from the negative syndrome. Keshavan et al. (1988) found that such patients were more likely than other schizophrenic patients to have abnormal dexamethasone and thyrotropin-releasing hormone tests. Owen et al. (1989a) showed that lateral ventricular enlargement on computed tomography (CT) was found in those schizophrenic patients with no family history and in those with a family history of schizophrenia, but not in those with a family history of affective disorder.

The Kraepelinian basis for the dichotomy between schizophrenia and affective disorder was that the former showed a worse outcome, with lack of full recovery between episodes (largely due to persisting negative symptoms), whereas affective disorder showed a propensity to remit. It may be that these longitudinal features, in effect the presence or absence of negative symptoms, are a central part of the heritable element in schizophrenia. This view is supported by the observed familial link between schizophrenia and a group of non-psychotic, enduring abnormalities of affect, speech, thought, and social functioning (i.e., the schizophrenia spectrum in general and schizotypal personality disorder in particular). Several authors have pointed to the similarity between the diagnostic criteria for residual schizophrenia and those for schizotypal disorder. A working hypothesis (Kendler 1985) might be that the true phenotype in schizophrenia comprises a syndrome of negative symptoms; the patient would present as schizophrenia if supplemented by positive symptoms, as schizotypal disorder if not.

The recent molecular genetic study of Sherrington et al. (1988) revealed that the likelihood of linkage to two probes on the proximal long arm of chromosome 5 in the seven multiply affected families studied was higher when not only schizophrenic and spectrum individuals were considered as cases, but when "fringe" cases were also counted as affected. This finding also suggests that it is not schizophrenia that is inherited per se, but a predisposition to a wider range of psychiatric abnormalities. If this study is confirmed, it will be important to establish whether the cases regarded as fringe have negative symptoms.

Overall, the evidence is that negative features are more heritable than positive symptoms. Features like lack of social functioning and cognitive deficits can antedate the development of a positive picture or occur in those relatives of schizophrenic patients who never develop positive symptoms.

ORGANIC ENVIRONMENTAL FACTORS

Only a minority of individuals who develop schizophrenia have a similarly affected relative. One cannot assume that apparently "sporadic" cases do not have a genetic etiology, but there is increasing evidence that environmental factors can interact with or replace genetic factors in causing schizophrenia. The first distinction to make in this context is that environmentally mediated organic factors should be clearly distinguished from environmentally situated psychosocial factors.

Organic brain diseases play an etiologic role in a small subgroup of "sporadic" schizophrenias (Davison and Bagley 1969). The best-studied example is schizophrenia arising in the context of temporal lobe epilepsy. Many authors have noted that whereas the positive symptoms found in such cases are indistinguishable from Schneiderian first-rank symptoms, negative symptoms are uncommon (McKenna et al. 1985; Perez and Trimble 1980; Toone et al. 1982). Indeed, Trimble (1990), extrapolating from his studies of psychotic patients with temporal lobe epilepsy, advanced the view that first-rank symptoms are a manifestation of temporal lobe dysfunction. Impaired premorbid personality also seems rarer in epileptic schizophrenic psychoses, and Slater et al. (1963) noted that the minority of such patients with blunted affect had a significantly earlier age of onset.

A similar observation was made by Davison and Bagley (1969), who noted that negative features such as affective blunting and incongruity characterized those secondary schizophrenias in which there was a relatively early onset of the central nervous system disorder and the psychosis. The importance of the timing of the cerebral lesion in the pathogenesis of secondary schizophrenias has been reiterated (Weinberger 1987).

Neuroimaging techniques have re-invigorated the search for organic antecedents in schizophrenia. CT findings of lateral and third ventricular enlargement and cortical sulcal widening in some schizophrenic patients compared to healthy controls are being replicated. The weight of evidence suggests that these radiologic abnormalities reflect a long-standing, static lesion rather than the progressive atrophy of a neurodegenerative disorder (Murray and Lewis 1987). The abnormalities do not progress on follow-up, are found in young patients in their first episode, and are not clearly correlated with length of illness or treatment (Lewis 1989). By implication, the structural brain abnormalities seen on CT predate the onset of the psychosis and may signal the neuropathologic sequelae of etiologic events earlier, perhaps much earlier, in life.

Attempts to identify clinical correlates of CT abnormalities in schizophrenia have centered on the most-studied finding of lateral ventricular enlargement. Using statistically derived cutoff points to define such enlargement, typically two or more standard deviations above the control mean, several groups have found cognitive impairment on objective testing (Goldberg and Weinberger 1986; Owens et al. 1985). A history of poor premorbid adjustment has also been found by some studies to correlate with ventricular enlargement (Weinberger et al. 1980a; Williams et al. 1985). Since clinical studies have revealed fairly consistent links between these two measures and the presence of negative symptoms, it might reasonably be expected that an association between negative symptoms and ventricular enlargement would emerge. Despite earlier claims, however, the evidence is conflicting, with roughly equal numbers of studies finding the presence and absence of such an association (Crow 1985).

More recently, associations have been sought between ventricular enlargement and etiologic risk factors for schizophrenia. The best-established etiologic marker is a manifest family history. Our interpretation of the evidence (Lewis et al. 1987; Murray et al. 1985) is that an inverse correlation exists between morbid risk to relatives and ventricular enlargement; that is, ventricular enlargement largely characterizes "sporadic" schizophrenia. By no means have all studies demonstrated this association, however, and as noted above, we recently found that normal ventricles were confined specifically to schizophrenic patients with a family history of affective disorder (Owen et al. 1989a).

Since ventricular enlargement does not seem to be a product of a genetic diathesis, it presumably reflects the action of some organic environmental factor. Certainly, there are such factors that can both increase the risk of schizophrenia and are also capable of giving rise to nonprogressive CT changes such as ventricular enlargement. Examples include head injury and encephalitis.

Another class of early environmental organic insults known to lead to nonprogressive ventricular and sulcal enlargement are those arising in the pre- and perinatal period (Lewis et al. 1989; Murray et al. 1985). Furthermore, prematurity, oxygen deprivation during labor (and also in utero), and viral infections during pregnancy have all been implicated in the cause of schizophrenia (Jacobsen and Kinney 1980; McNeil 1988; Mednick et al. 1988). The evidence is that such obstetric complications confer about a twofold relative risk for the disorder (Goodman 1988; Lewis 1989).

Support for this view comes from recent postmortem studies of schizophrenic patients, which have shown not only enlarged ventricles and decreased volume of hippocampus, parahippocampal gyrus, amygdala, and internal pallidum (Bogerts et al. 1985; Brown et al. 1986), but also cytoarchitectural abnormalities consistent with dysplasia due to pre- or perinatal disturbance of neurodevelopment (Jakob and Beckmann 1986; Kovelman and Scheibel 1984).

Unfortunately, few investigators have examined the characteristics of those schizophrenias consequent to obstetric complications. Owen et al. (1989b), however, found an association of obstetric complications with male sex, earlier onset, poor premorbid personality, and enlarged ventricles, all features that have been associated with negative symptoms.

PSYCHOSOCIAL ENVIRONMENT

The other class of environmental factors that have been studied extensively as potential risk factors for schizophrenia is psychosocial in nature. Broadly, it includes factors in the existential environment that have the potential to confer psychological "stress," on the one hand, or result in psychological "understimulation" on the other.

The capacity of overly regulated environments to exacerbate certain types of negative symptoms such as withdrawal, poverty of speech, and anhedonia was established in the classic studies of institutional care by Wing and Brown (1970). The practical importance of these studies was immense. They have become a cornerstone of social intervention and rehabilitation programs. Yet factors such as an understimulating environment are clearly sources of secondary rather than primary disability. Overregimented institutional care compounds rather than causes negative symptoms. Furthermore, Brown and Wing also demonstrated that an overstimulating psychosocial environment could cause the reemergence or worsening of positive symptoms. The study of life events around the onset of first or subsequent episodes of schizophrenia arose in parallel with this work (Brown and Birley 1968), but the number of well-conducted studies is still small. The largest is that to emerge from the World Health Organization multicenter collaborative study (Day et al. 1987), in which 386 patients were screened for the occurrence of independent life events prior to the onset of psychosis. Overall, the results suggested an increase in life events in the 3-week period prior to onset, the same as the period found in the original Brown and Birley (1968) study.

Life events research in schizophrenia (Leff et al. 1973) must be judged in the context of two thorny issues: specificity and causality. An increase in life events has been demonstrated prior to the onset of several psychiatric and general medical disorders, and the link in schizophrenia is not as strong as it may be for the onset of affective disorders. Furthermore, a distinction must be made between genuine causation of positive symptoms (the symptoms would never have occurred in the absence of the event) and mere precipitation (the symptoms depend on the event only for their timing, not their occurrence per se). Most authors would now agree that life events operate as nonspecific triggers for the onset of positive symptoms rather than as specific etiologic risk factors (Leff 1987).

Similar caveats of specificity and causality operate for the particular form of more chronic psychosocial stress termed *high expressed emotion*. Several studies have demonstrated that in patients with established schizophrenia, positive symptoms are more likely to emerge in the presence of domestic criticism, hostility, and emotional overinvolvement (Leff and Vaughn 1985). Recently, however, skepticism has arisen about the construct validity of the measure, and some groups have pointed to the importance of previous chronicity (MacMillan et al. 1987) and extraneous variables such as gender and prognosis (Hogarty 1985) in explaining the link between relapse rate and high expressed emotion. It seems likely that cause-effect relationships are reciprocal in this area: the presence of chronic negative symptoms may elevate expressed emotion, resulting in an exacerbation of positive symptoms.

Thus the evidence is strong that psychosocial-environmental stressors can trigger or exacerbate positive symptoms, and that an environment abnormally devoid of such stressors (such as a long-stay hospital ward) can exacerbate certain negative symptoms. There is no conclusive evidence that either condition is truly causative of either type of syndrome.

A DEVELOPMENTAL VIEW

Although negative symptoms can be exacerbated by certain social environments, they appear to be more fundamentally associated with poor premorbid adjustment and educational achievement. Kay et al. (1986b) point out that this observation raises the possibility of pre-existing developmental failures. Indeed, most of the other features proposed by Crow (1980a, 1985) as characterizing the Type II syndrome (cognitive impairment, poor social functioning, ventricular enlargement, neurologic soft signs) have been reported to be present before the onset of positive symptoms in adult life. We consider, therefore, that the negative syndrome is best explained by a developmental model of schizophrenia (Lewis 1989; Murray et al. 1988).

Table 12-3 shows a preliminary analysis of data from our current study of etiologic and developmental variables in 95 patients admitted to the Maudsley Hospital with functional psychosis (56 with DSM-III schizophrenia and schizophreniform disorder, 38 with affective psychosis, and one with atypical psychosis). Negative symptoms (self-neglect and blunted affect), as measured by the Present State Examination (Wing et al. 1974) during the episode, showed a significant correlation with residual negative symptoms following first admission, as rated by an interview with the patient's mother. In the schizophrenic patients, negative symptoms during the episode correlated more highly with a family history of affective disorder than with a family history of schizophrenia or a history of obstetric complications. This runs counter to the findings of Kendler and Tsuang (1988). It may be that our ratings reflect symptoms that are predominantly state related and are in part a manifestation of depression.

Residual negative symptoms were significantly correlated with residual positive symptoms, indicating the tendency of patients who do not wholly recover to show both types of symptoms. Both types of residual symptoms were positively correlated with a history of obstetric complications, indicating an association between obstetric complications and severity and chronicity. Patients who had a history of developmental problems (e.g., poor language development or

Table 12-3. Correlation of symptoms and risk factors in 95 patients with functional psychosis

	Negative residual symptoms[b]	Positive residual symptoms[b]	Birth weight	Obstetric complications[c]	Family history of schizophrenia[d]	Family history of major depression[d]
Negative symptoms[a]	.39*** (.44***)	.20 (.25)	-.05 (-.01)	.13 (.09)	.04 (.09)	.04 (.24*)
Negative residual symptoms[b]		.67*** (.64***)	-.32** (-.25)	.38*** (.25)	.12 (.01)	.03 (.05)
Positive residual symptoms[b]			-.16 (-.11)	.44*** (.44**)	.20 (.16)	.02 (-.05)
Birth weight				-.29** (-.34**)	-.12 (.03)	.23* (.25)
Obstetric complications[c]					-.10 (-.18)	-.02 (-.01)
Family history of schizophrenia[d]						-.03 (.05)
Family history of major depression[d]						

Note. Correlations for the 56 schizophrenic patients are given in parentheses.
[a]Blunted affect and self-neglect. [b]Following first admission. [c]Defined according to Lewis et al. (1989). [d]In first-degree relatives.
*$P < .05$. **$P < .01$. ***$P < .001$.

enuresis) had a significantly lower birth weight than those without such problems; patients with either low birth weight or a family history of schizophrenia had a poorer premorbid adjustment than those who lacked either of these two risk factors.

A variety of environmental factors can impair brain development during fetal and neonatal life, and, as we anticipated, a history of obstetric complications correlated both with poor premorbid adjustment and with residual negative symptoms. They also predicted residual positive symptoms, presumably indicating that a history of obstetric complications is associated with a relatively severe form of schizophrenia.

In our sample, a family history of schizophrenia correlated with poor premorbid adjustment but not significantly with negative symptoms. This finding, however, may be a consequence of the relatively small size of the sample; there is ample evidence, as we noted earlier, that genetic factors contribute to negative symptoms. In a related study, Cannon et al. (1990) observed that among a group of 138 individuals at high risk for developing schizophrenia, those at elevated genetic risk who suffered severe delivery complications were significantly more likely to evidence outcomes of schizophrenia with predominantly negative symptoms. This finding highlights the importance of genetic-environmental interactions in the production of negative symptoms.

It warrants repeating that the majority of schizophrenic patients have no history of a similarly affected relative, or of obstetric complications or other potential cerebral insults. We do not know whether they carry predisposing genes or subtle and as yet undetectable brain damage. The manifest presence in the history of certain environmental or genetic risk factors, however, appears to exert not only a pathogenic but also a pathoplastic effect on schizophrenic symptoms. The severity and admixture of positive and negative symptoms, as well as the timing of onset and course, do seem to be influenced by such risk factors, although our understanding of the mechanisms is still crude. This picture is entirely consistent with the formulation of schizophrenia as a syndrome—that is, a collection of symptoms, none of which in isolation is pathognomonic—that can arise from a variety of underlying causes.

Treatment

Chapter 13

Therapeutic Approaches to Negative Symptoms

William T. Carpenter, Jr., M.D.
Robert R. Conley, M.D.

Chapter 13

Therapeutic Approaches to Negative Symptoms

Although negative symptoms constitute the most debilitating component of schizophrenic psychopathology, their underlying pathophysiologic basis is poorly understood. As a consequence, treatment strategies based on empirical findings in clinical trials and on an understanding of pathophysiology have not been developed. Present therapeutic approaches to negative symptoms are principally dependent on assumptions about the cause of the negative symptoms. Despite these limitations, there are several therapeutic techniques that can be welded into an individual effective treatment program.

Negative symptoms constitute a discrete domain of schizophrenic psychopathology (primary) (Carpenter and Buchanan 1989). They may also occur as a consequence of a range of other factors in schizophrenia; such secondary negative symptoms are usually responsive to treatment of the underlying cause. The first step in the treatment of negative symptoms is to distinguish between primary and secondary negative symptoms and, if the latter, to treat the underlying cause.

In the treatment of schizophrenic patients, focusing attention mainly on positive symptoms and bizarre behavior has led to frustration and misunderstanding among patients and family members. Negative symptoms often cause the greatest difficulties with daily functioning and interacting with others, yet they are often considered by caretakers, families, and patients themselves as simply unattractive personality characteristics. Careful distinction of primary from secondary negative symptoms is critical; correct identification of the latter can lead to efficacious treatment and an improvement in life functioning. An example of this possibility is the change seen in a previously poorly responsive patient who improved markedly with clozapine

Supported in part by NIMH grants MH-40279, MH-35996, and MH-09044.

207

therapy. His illness included marked negative symptoms. With effective treatment of his core psychosis, it was seen that, although he continued to show a restricted emotional range, the symptoms of apathy, anhedonia, and lack of purpose abated. It gradually became apparent that these symptoms were related to a demoralized state. Careful counseling of the patient and his family was needed for them to appreciate this change, however, as superficially the patient did not seem markedly improved. Once the patient and his support network felt optimistic about his capacity for change, rehabilitation was enhanced. The patient now works full-time and is living semi-independently. The primary negative symptom of restricted emotional range persists, but the abatement of psychosis and the secondary negative symptoms allows significant social and occupational functioning.

TREATMENT OF SECONDARY NEGATIVE SYMPTOMS

Negative symptoms (Strauss et al. 1974) is a generically descriptive term for various manifestations of diminished capacity for ordinary behavioral functioning (see Carpenter et al., Chapter 1, this volume). Putative negative symptoms include apathy, anhedonia, restricted emotional arousal, reduced volition and motivation, diminished social drive, and lack of a sense of purpose. Such symptom manifestations are known to be associated with drug effects, dysphoric mood, understimulating environments, and demoralization. They are often observed during periods of intense psychosis and have sometimes been hypothesized to represent adaptive responses aimed at diminishing information overload and sensory stimulation. The rational treatment of negative symptoms requires a careful differentiation of those secondary to the above factors from those that constitute enduring primary or deficit symptoms. As secondary reactions, these negative symptoms can be expected to fluctuate in association with the underlying cause.

Briefly summarized, when negative symptoms are observed in the context of florid psychosis, the initial task is the treatment of psychosis per se with neuroleptics, reduction of stimulation, and supportive therapy. If this condition is effectively treated, negative symptoms may abate and not require special therapeutic consideration. As discussed in other chapters and amply demonstrated in other publications, negative as well as positive symptoms often improve in response to antipsychotic drugs.

Negative symptoms that do not abate may actually be neuroleptic adverse effects. Akinesia is a prime example of a symptom that is easily mistaken for restricted affective expression in the schizophrenic patient. Drug-induced negative symptoms can be treated by changing to a neuroleptic with a different side effect profile, by decreasing dosage, by discontinuing medication and using a targeted intervention approach, by substituting an atypical antipsychotic medication, or by using anticholinergic antiparkinsonian drugs.

During periods of relative remission or stability of psychosis, patients may experience dysphoric mood states. Anyone with intense anxiety or depression will exhibit secondary negative symptoms such as anhedonia. If a mood disturbance is suspected as the cause of negative symptoms, a direct therapeutic approach to the mood disturbance may be required using antidepressants (Siris et al. 1987) or anxiolytics (Csernansky et al. 1984); psychotherapy may be necessary. A range of interpersonal and pharmacologic techniques is thus available to the clinician for integration into the therapeutic strategy.

The problem of dealing with negative symptoms when they are associated with demoralization is a difficult one. Little is known about what constitutes effective therapeutic intervention for persevering demoralization. A highly individualized approach predicated on an understanding of the reasons for demoralization and the patient's responsiveness to various supportive measures appears warranted.

Many long-term hospital and community-based patients live in under-stimulating environments. The supposition that environmental deprivation produces or contributes to negative symptoms is more speculative. It draws on a literature relating chronicity to custodial care and to the general effects of social and intellectual isolation. Although applications will vary, therapeutic approaches will seek relevant environmental enhancement for patients whose negative symptoms are associated with living in circumstances of exceptional isolation. Since it is known that overstimulation and "social push" therapies can exacerbate symptoms in some patients, the strategy would be to move gradually toward optimal levels of stimulation, avoiding excessive or stressful stimulation.

In the above paragraphs, we have touched on known or suspected causes for secondary negative symptoms observed in patients with schizophrenia. With the exception of the extrapyramidal side effects of neuroleptic drugs, there is little specific information that is available from clinical trials relevant to the treatment of negative symptoms. There is not yet a substantial body of work on the reliability and validity of differential diagnoses of negative symptoms, but preliminary work is encouraging (Buchanan et al., unpublished data; Carpenter et al. 1988; Chapman and Chapman 1985; Kirkpatrick et al., unpublished data; Thaker et al. 1988; Wagman et al. 1987). Clinicians routinely face the challenge of ascertaining whether negative symptoms are present in a given schizophrenic patient, and if so, the likely cause. Since many causes are treatable, it is crucial that the challenge of differential diagnosis be accepted and that clinicians be prepared to implement treatment, even in the absence of definitive evidence for a specific etiologic factor. There is good reason to proceed since the approaches in question are generally safe and follow well-established clinical rationales.

The more difficult task is that of treating primary negative symptoms of schizophrenia, the constellation that has been the major focus of this volume.

TREATMENT OF PRIMARY NEGATIVE SYMPTOMS

Primary negative symptoms can be subdivided into transitory and enduring, or state and trait, pathologic features. There are few empirical data that specifically address treatment of primary negative symptoms. In both the descriptive literature and in clinical trials, inferences regarding negative symptom therapeutics have been limited by two major problems. First, the distinction between primary and secondary symptoms is not made, leaving undetermined the extent to which clinical improvement reflects a lessening of primary pathology. Second, the distinction between state and trait psychopathology is not generally made.

Recognizing these limitations, we now discuss specific pharmacologic and psychiatric rehabilitation strategies for the treatment of primary negative symptoms.

Pharmacotherapy

Negative symptoms are known to decrease during effective treatment of psychosis (Goldberg 1985). The time course of improvement roughly corresponds to the time course of improvement in the positive symptom domain, suggesting either a secondary response to treatment of psychosis, a similar mode of therapeutic efficacy, or related underlying mechanisms. On the other hand, it is generally observed that clinically stable patients with long-standing deficits fail to have a robust (negative symptom) response to neuroleptic medication (Angst 1988; Bleuler 1978; Carpenter and Kirkpatrick 1988; Ciompi 1980; Harding 1988; Huber 1980; McGlashan and Carpenter 1988). These findings, taken together, suggest that whereas nonenduring (primary or secondary) negative symptoms may improve with neuroleptic treatment, enduring or deficit primary negative symptoms may not be responsive to neuroleptics. Parenthetically, a study designed to isolate a therapeutic effect on primary negative symptoms would have to assess treatment effect during a period in which psychosis is either remitted or stable. Contemporaneous effects are always difficult to interpret.

Of particular interest in the pharmacotherapy of primary negative symptoms are the results of a multicenter clozapine study (Kane et al. 1988). In this study, chronically psychotic patients, well-defined as neuroleptic nonresponders, proved more responsive to clozapine than to chlorpromazine during a 6-week trial. This difference emerged both in a positive symptom factor and in a negative symptom factor comprising restricted affect and several proxy measures. It is noteworthy that the effect of clozapine on negative symptoms appeared to be more robust than that on positive symptoms, making it unlikely that the observed treatment effect was solely secondary to the reduction of psychosis. Since stable patients often improve on this factor during drug discontinuation, however, it is possible that a diminution of side effects was partially responsible for the superiority of clozapine in the putative negative symptom domain. Far more interesting is the possibility that differences in mechanisms of action of typical and atypical neuroleptics translate into a different profile of therapeutic efficacy. Clozapine's antiserotonergic activity, potent anticholinergic property, and its different D_1 and D_2 dopamine receptor affinities (Farde et al. 1987, 1990) as compared to other neuroleptics have been involved to explain its therapeutic effect on negative symptoms. A better understanding of the pharmacologic basis of clozapine's greater efficacy in ameliorating negative symptoms would aid in the development of more effective agents to treat negative symptoms.

Other agents such as anticholinergics, benzodiazepines, and propranolol have also been employed in the treatment of negative symptoms. The rationale for their use and their efficacy are discussed elsewhere (Meltzer, Chapter 14, this volume).

Psychiatric Rehabilitation

The loss of functional skills has been considered a primary pathogenic process in schizophrenia, and even as a diagnostic criterion (Andreasen 1985). Recovery of these skills, however, has been neglected in the focus on the treatment of positive symptoms. The relative refractoriness of negative symptoms to conventional treatment of schizophrenia has fueled the development of a variety of psychiatric rehabilitation strategies. Rehabilitation interventions are aimed at 1) building social, vocational, cognitive, and other skills in the patient; and 2) providing supportive and "prosthetic" environments in an effort to minimize the impact of the "deficit" symptoms on the patient's adaptational capacity.

Skills training attempts to improve the patient's functioning through a variety of psychological (chiefly behavioral) treatments. These interventions should be closely linked to initial and ongoing assessments of the patient. The first step involves an assessment of the patient's social adaptation prior to the onset of the illness. This assessment should include an evaluation of the patient's intellectual potential in education and occupation, stability of the patient's interpersonal relationships, emotional involvement and stability, and the patient's acceptance of general principles that guide interpersonal behavior. Using this framework, the patient's current competence and skill should next be assessed in terms of the stresses and expectations of social and family life and employment that the patient will have to encounter. Based on this evaluation, "target" deficits are identified and attempts to train (or retrain) the patient to correct these deficits are initiated. For skills training to be effective, it is not sufficient to determine that a deficit exists; the patient must perceive this deficit and be motivated to do something about it. A number of specific (Doane et al. 1985; Falloon and Liberman 1983; Falloon and Pederson 1985; Falloon et al. 1985; Liberman and Evans 1985; Liberman and Mueser 1989; Liberman et al. 1985; May et al. 1985; Wallace and Liberman 1985) and general (Alanen et al. 1985; Brenner 1989; Lindberg 1981) approaches have been described and their efficacy evaluated.

Since there are many similarities between deficit symptoms and features of frontal lobe dysfunction, principles of frontal lobe training may be applicable (Craine 1982; Luria 1973, 1974). Relevant principles include: 1) problem-solving strategies to encourage stepwise solutions to complex tasks; 2) development of communication skills using a behavioral paradigm and articulated feedback; 3) exercises to improve verbal fluency; 4) exercises to improve intellectual flexibility and ability to change sets; and 5) exercises to help patients analyze the consequences of various behaviors so that they can better regulate that behavior and avoid counterproductive behavior.

Multi-task groups are usually an effective treatment modality; patients generally adapt well to a "parallel play" mode of group structure. Therapy that involves specific life skills, such as money management, interpersonal relations, and job skills, is better tolerated in general than less-focused task groups. For example, a planned group meal will allow individual work in money management, motor skills, life skills, and interpersonal relations if the tasks of budgeting, shopping, preparing, and serving are distributed among patients with different skills and needs (McDermott and Conley 1986; Prien 1980). Social skills training in a behavioral therapy model that emphasizes the individuality of each patient has been shown to be efficacious. It allows patients to model the behavior of peers who have skills in areas in which they themselves are lacking, while they, in turn, can serve as models in their own areas of strength. Again, careful attention to allowing patients to succeed and minimizing frustration and embarrassment is critical for success.

Since many patients have limited potential for acquiring and generalizing functional skills sufficient for independent living, however, it is important to develop and maintain long-term support systems that will preserve functioning and minimize deterioration despite the presence of chronic disabilities that cannot be successfully treated. Such environmental "prostheses" include supervised residential and vocational settings, day hospitals and day centers, and case management. The availability of effective community support is critical. To this end, the development of peer support groups and family networks targeted toward the severely mentally ill is encouraging. It is also helpful to note that, in several states, patients discharged from state hospitals must be placed in an approved living situation where therapy and rehabilitation are available. As communities become better educated to the possibility of change in patients, more change will be seen.

Although a discussion of these specific techniques is beyond the scope of this chapter (and detailed discussions are available, e.g., in *Schizophrenia Bulletin* 1986, Volume 12, No. 4, entire issue), we wish to emphasize some general principles.

First, although patients with primary enduring or deficit symptoms share many characteristics that define the range of therapeutic considerations, the actual selection and implementation of treatment in any given case must depend on the specific evaluations of the individual patient and his or her circumstances. Such individualized decision making requires a strong and continuous clinical relationship in which the clinician must be intimately informed about the patient's inner world, reactivity to various environmental circumstances, and responsiveness to various therapeutic maneuvers. It is therefore important to provide an environment in which routines are relaxed, depersonalization is avoided, and the social distance between patient and staff is reduced; "block" treatments with all patients doing the same thing at the same time should be avoided.

Second, it must be recognized that deficit symptoms are associated with chronic, persistent disability; consequently the rehabilitation process needs to be continuous or repetitive. This would obviously create problems if mental health services were funded on the basis of "single-episode" users. Even in the absence of financial problems, maintaining staff morale in the face of "little apparent progress" could be difficult. Furthermore, in view of the fluctuating nature of schizophrenic illness, the patient's adaptive capacity is bound to be unstable and changing.

Third, although patients often have functional deficits in multiple areas, rehabilitation should first address those areas in which the patient seems most capable of progress. As the patient begins to have successes, more challenging areas can be addressed. If a treatment goal proves too frustrating to a patient, it should be de-emphasized and replaced with another task. In this way, areas in which improvement may be possible are explored serially as treatment progresses. Patients make gains where they are capable of improving, while frustration is minimized, particularly at early stages of treatment.

Fourth, data from long-term follow-up studies suggest that diminution of psychosis and improved social and occupational performance are frequently associated with increased age (Angst 1988; Bleuler 1978; Carpenter and Kirkpatrick 1988; Ciompi 1980; Harding 1988; Huber et al. 1980; McGlashan and Carpenter 1988). Reducing drug side effects and implementing rehabilitative procedures may be especially effective in this phase of illness. The elderly patient requires special rehabilitative programming. We have found such patients to be particularly interested in techniques for comfortably dealing with family members. Affect is often difficult to express, and emotion in others may be confusing. The issue of respect is often a prominent factor in demoralization. Patients with chronic schizophrenia often feel removed from their appropriate place in the family hierarchy. They feel infantilized by family members and caretakers. Often positive and negative symptoms are equated with dementia (Borson et al. 1987). The particular demands of therapeutics and rehabilitation of aging patients with schizophrenia should be a priority area for research, because there is currently a dearth of empirical data.

CONCLUSIONS

Treatment of negative symptoms is just beginning to be explored. At present, the key is to distinguish primary from secondary negative symptoms, which are generally responsive to available treatments. Primary, enduring negative (deficit) symptoms are minimally responsive to present therapy. Atypical neuroleptics and drugs active in cholinergic, adrenergic, and serotonergic systems are being explored for treatment relevance. Cognitive, occupational, and social rehabilitation procedures offer rational approaches to the schizophrenia deficit.

Chapter 14

Pharmacologic Treatment of Negative Symptoms

Herbert Y. Meltzer, M.D.

Chapter 14

Pharmacologic Treatment of Negative Symptoms

The development of effective pharmacologic treatments for the negative symptoms of schizophrenia has become a major objective in recent years (Meltzer, in press; Meltzer et al. 1986). This was not always the case. As discussed elsewhere (Meltzer, in press), the major goal of new antipsychotic drug development until the 1980s was the treatment of positive symptoms (e.g. delusions, hallucinations, and some types of thought disorder). Interest in the issue of treating negative symptoms was heightened by the provocative suggestion of Crow (1980a) that negative symptoms in chronic schizophrenic patients were insensitive to neuroleptic treatment. This conclusion was based mainly on the study of Johnstone et al. (1978b), which found that *cis*-flupentixol, an effective dopamine receptor blocker, had no greater effect on negative symptoms than *trans*-flupentixol, an isomer of *cis*-flupentixol, which lacks dopamine antagonist properties. Furthermore, Crow (1980a) argued that a syndrome of schizophrenia characterized by predominant negative symptoms (Type II) might be irreversible, in part because it could be due to structural abnormalities of the brain. Crow (1980a) suggested that functional changes in the dopaminergic system were the basis of the more neuroleptic-responsive positive symptoms that were predominant in the so-called Type I syndrome.

The ethos of deinstitutionalization in the United States in the 1960s and 1970s led to the discharge of nearly two-thirds of all chronically hospitalized schizophrenic patients and to a marked reluctance toward indefinite hospitalizations of relapsing schizophrenic patients. These changes in clinical practice made the ability to treat

Supported by in part by NIMH grant numbers MH-41684 and MH-41683, and grants from the Cleveland Foundation, The Sawyer Foundation, and The Laureate Foundation (NARSAD). Dr. Meltzer is the recipient of NIMH Research Scientist Award MH-47808.

217

negative symptoms of even greater importance. Hospital administrators and public health officials, interested in having as many schizophrenic patients as possible leave their institutions, became sensitized to the need to develop better pharmacologic treatment of negative symptoms. Negative symptoms such as withdrawal, lack of motivation, blunted affect, and motor retardation are much more detrimental to the functioning of a schizophrenic patient in the community, where self-reliance is more essential than for a hospitalized patient. In the community, where only family members or few clinically trained people are available to help meet various needs, negative symptoms may cause even more disability and suffering than positive symptoms.

The purpose of this chapter will be to consider some of the major issues concerning the pharmacologic treatment of negative symptoms and to review the evidence concerning the effect of neuroleptic and other antipsychotic drugs on negative symptoms.

CONCEPTUAL ISSUES

Accurate assessment is the first step in the consideration of whether antipsychotic drugs affect negative symptoms. Virtually all prospective or retrospective studies of negative symptoms have utilized broad-based rating scales that include a small number of items generally considered to be negative in nature—for example, the Krawiecka-Manchester Scale (Krawiecka et al. 1977), the Brief Psychiatric Rating Scale (BPRS) (Overall and Gorham 1962), and the Comprehensive Psychiatric Rating Scale (Asberg et al. 1978). The negative symptoms subscales embedded in these instruments make no pretense to be comprehensive. Nevertheless, they have been found to be responsive to drug treatment. More comprehensive negative symptom scales, such as the Scale for the Assessment of Negative Symptoms (Andreasen 1983), were not designed for pharmacologic studies and need to be shown to be sensitive to drug-induced changes. The Abrams and Taylor Scale for Emotional Bunting (Abrams and Taylor 1978) was found to show responses comparable to those of the BPRS negative symptoms cluster following withdrawal and administration of neuroleptic drugs (Breier 1987). The Positive and Negative Syndrome Scale (PANSS) (Kay et al. 1987a, 1987b), the Negative Symptom Rating Scale (Iager et al. 1985), and the Negative Symptom Assessment (Alphs and Summerfelt 1989) are specifically designed for negative symptoms but they have not yet been demonstrated to be useful in clinical drug trials, with the exception of the PANSS (Feinberg et al. 1988). Rating scales are reviewed in greater detail elsewhere (Silk and Tandon, Chapter 4, this volume).

Little consideration has been given to the possibility of using changes in social function, which would appear to be closely related to negative symptoms, as a dependent variable reflecting negative symptoms. However, such an approach would be consistent with the view of Strauss et al. (1974) that these symptoms are a critical component of the deficit state, which is a core aspect of schizophrenia. These authors distinguished primary negative symptoms such as anhedonia and loss of motivation from the secondary negative symptoms such as slowed movement secondary to neuroleptic-induced parkinsonism or apathy due to institutionalization in a custodial environment. Although such distinctions are of great importance, they may be quite difficult to make in many research situations.

Because the major focus of virtually all clinical drug trials has been on the relatively easily measured positive symptoms such as delusions and hallucinations, it is possible that neuroleptic-induced improvement in negative symptoms in previous studies went unnoted. Even more likely is the possibility that the time course of improvement in negative symptoms is slower than that of positive symptoms. Therefore, the early studies of neuroleptic efficacy, usually of 4 weeks' duration, in chronic schizophrenic patients with an acute exacerbation may have been too short to demonstrate an improvement in negative symptoms that might not have occurred until several months later. The major effect of antipsychotic drugs on negative symptoms could be an interaction with a variety of psychosocial therapies that are themselves ineffective or minimally effective (Falloon and Liberman 1983; Mosher and Meltzer 1980). Such therapies may be under-represented or even deliberately restricted in acute drug trials. Such an interaction might be dependent on an outpatient environment. This may account for some of the apparent advantages of pimozide and related drugs in treating negative symptoms, as will be discussed subsequently.

The effectiveness of antipsychotic drugs to diminish negative symptoms may also be restricted to specific subtypes of schizophrenia, and may be a function of duration of illness, the number of previous psychotic exacerbations, severity of illness, or the stage of the evolution of the schizophrenic process. The heterogeneity in the etiology of schizophrenia is a well-accepted, if unproven, postulate (Meltzer 1979). Even if the concept of Type I and II schizophrenia (Crow 1980a) has limited validity (Meltzer 1985), it is possible that negative symptoms in subtypes (such as paranoid or undifferentiated, good versus poor premorbid) may respond differently to neuroleptic drug treatment. A better effect of neuroleptic treatment on negative symptoms might be expected in the earlier stages of the illness. There is evidence that dopaminergic function may decrease with duration of illness (Meltzer et al. 1984) and that decreased dopaminergic activity may be related to the etiology of negative symptoms (Meltzer 1987). Negative symptoms are usually treated as a unitary concept; that is, there is an expectation that antipsychotic drugs should be effective against the full spectrum of negative symptoms for a specific patient or for a group of patients. However, there may be heterogeneity in the responsiveness of specific negative symptoms to neuroleptic drugs based on differences in the etiology of symptoms such as lack of motivation and withdrawal, as well as individual differences in the etiology of specific negative symptoms. For these reasons, heterogeneity in the outcome of the effect of antipsychotic drug treatment on negative symptoms is to be expected.

The issue of the relationship between improvement in negative symptoms as a function of improvement in positive symptoms or improvement in negative symptoms in patients who have little or no positive symptoms versus those with high levels of positive symptoms is one that requires specific attention (Meltzer 1985). It may be that the effect of treatment on negative symptoms is dependent on positive symptom improvement and would therefore be less in schizophrenic patients with either few positive symptoms or with positive symptoms resistant to neuroleptic drugs.

EFFECT OF NEUROLEPTIC DRUGS ON NEGATIVE SYMPTOMS

Cole et al. (1966) reviewed five early, large-scale, placebo-controlled studies (Casey et al. 1960a, 1960b; Gorham and Polorny 1964; Klein 1967; Kurland et al. 1961) that considered the effect of neuroleptic drugs on negative symptoms. Two of the five studies showed greater improvement in blunted affect and indifference with neuroleptic treatment and four showed a positive effect on withdrawal and retardation.

We have reviewed in detail elsewhere (Meltzer et al. 1986) the results of the National Institute of Mental Health (1964, 1967) Psychopharmacology Service Center collaborative studies (Goldberg et al. 1965), which were among the first to address the responsiveness of negative symptoms to neuroleptic treatment and schizophrenia. In brief, these studies involved a double-blind, group comparison treatment of 344 relatively young, first admission schizophrenic patients treated with fluphenazine, chlorpromazine, thioridazine, or placebo for 6 weeks. In addition to improvement in positive symptoms, phenothiazine treatment was also associated with significantly greater improvement than placebo in the following negative symptoms: social participation, self-care, slowed speech and movements, indifference to the environment, and hebephrenic symptoms (blunted and inappropriate affect). Although lacking in the diagnostic rigor and close monitoring of interrater reliability expected of contemporary studies, this study strongly suggested a moderate effect of phenothiazine treatment on negative symptoms in relatively recent onset schizophrenic patients.

The issue of the effect of phenothiazine treatment as a function of duration of illness and dosage was addressed in several studies (Prien and Cole 1968; Prien et al. 1969). Negative symptoms such as retardation and apathy improved more in younger patients with briefer hospitalizations. Higher doses of phenothiazine (up to 2 g/day in chlorpromazine equivalents) were generally more effective in the younger patients. Negative symptoms also improved in some of the older patients with shorter periods of hospitalization, but generally with lower doses of phenothiazines. Older, chronically hospitalized patients tended to show the least improvement in both positive and negative symptoms. These studies suggest at least some effectiveness of neuroleptic drugs on negative symptoms in very chronic patients who were not preselected for very poor response to neuroleptic drugs. As will be discussed below, there is evidence that chronic schizophrenic patients selected for poor response of positive symptoms to neuroleptic drugs show little or no change in negative symptoms in response to haloperidol or chlorpromazine (Kane et al. 1988). Neuroleptics were also relatively ineffective in treating negative symptoms in the study of Serafetinides et al. (1972). The 57 chronic schizophrenic patients in this study were highly treatment resistant to neuroleptics with regard to positive symptoms. In another study that failed to find a consistent effect of chlorpromazine versus placebo on negative symptoms (Clark et al. 1963), the patient population also included chronically hospitalized schizophrenic patients.

As previously mentioned, Johnstone et al. (1978a) reported that *cis*-fluphentixol, an active dopamine receptor antagonist, was no more effective than *trans*-fluphentixol, its dopaminergically inactive isomer, or placebo in a double-blind trial of 45 acute schizophrenic patients. This study may be criticized on several grounds. The baseline ratings of negative symptoms were markedly different in the three treatment groups, but were still quite low in all groups. Such a floor effect mitigates against finding significant improvements in the negative symptoms. This study lasted for only 28 days and there were only 15 subjects in each group.

Meltzer (1985) reported a retrospective analysis of the effect of neuroleptic treatment, mainly with chlorpromazine or trifluoperazine on negative and positive symptoms in chronic schizophrenic patients diagnosed by Research Diagnostic Criteria (Spitzer et al. 1978). The negative symptoms were assessed by means of scales derived from the Schedule for Affective Disorders and Schizophrenia (SADS) (Endicott and Spitzer 1978). The negative symptom scale used in that study consisted of 11 items: blunted affect, inappropriate affect, poverty of content, loss of interest, loss of sexual interest, slowed speech, slow body movement, fatigue, incoherence, loose associations, and depressed appearance (Lewine et al. 1983). The positive symptoms scale consisted of 23 SADS items, all of which involve delusions and hallucinations. Total subscale scores were calculated by summing up items as absent or present. Significant differences in both positive and negative symptoms between pretreatment and discharge were observed. An analysis of covariance demonstrated that the decreases in positive symptoms and negative symptoms were significant even after covarying out the influence of the change in one from the change in the other. Improvement in this diverse group of negative symptoms was significantly greater in females than in males. Thus there was a 22% decrease in the negative symptom scale in male schizophrenic patients compared to a 40% decrease in female schizophrenic patients. At discharge, 35.5% (60/169) of the patients had negative symptom scale ratings of 0 or 1, compared to 59.2% (100/169) who had positive symptom scale ratings of 0 or 1, suggesting negative symptoms were more intransigent. Negative symptoms improved markedly in 38.2% (21/55) of the patients with marked negative symptoms at admission compared to marked improvement in positive symptoms in 56.4% (44/78) of the patients with marked positive symptoms at the beginning of treatment. Thus marked improvement in negative as well as positive symptoms was possible in this group, but such change was more common for positive symptoms.

This study may be criticized for including such items as inappropriate affect, incoherence, and loose associations as well as slowed speech, slowed body movement, and depressed appearance in a single negative symptom factor. The first group of symptoms have been found to be part of a separate factor, which we have labeled disorganization. This factor appears to be very sensitive to clozapine treatment. The second group of symptoms may be more closely related to depression, which may be either primary or secondary negative symptoms. Such items as blunted affect, withdrawal, and loss of interest form a third category of negative symptoms. These groupings do not necessarily emerge from factor analyses of large groups of candidate negative symptoms. Whether all three groups of symptoms should be considered to be negative symptoms is a moot point (Lewine and Sommers 1985; Sommers 1985).

We have recently reanalyzed these data using two separate negative subscales—one made of depressive-like items: loss of interest, slow speech, slow movement, and depressed appearance; and one made of disorganization items: inappropriate affect, poverty of thought content, incoherence, and loosening of associations. Blunted affect was examined separately. The positive symptom subscale was made up of the severity of hallucinations and severity of delusions items. For 77 schizophrenic patients treated with typical neuroleptic drugs, there were significant decreases in positive symptoms, negative depressive symptoms, and negative disorganization symptoms (Table 14-1). There was no significant change in blunted affect as a separate item (Table 14-1). Improvement in positive symptoms was still present after covarying out improvement in the other two scales or blunted affect. The improvement in the negative disorganization subscale was still significant after covarying out improvement in positive or negative depressive symptoms. The improvement in the negative depressive symptoms was present after covarying improvement in disorganization but not positive symptoms. These results indicate that some negative symptoms respond to neuroleptic treatment. Disorganization symptoms appear to respond independently of change in positive symptoms.

Breier et al. (1987) reported that negative symptoms increased slightly but significantly following a 4-week period of withdrawal of neuroleptic drugs in 19 young chronic schizophrenic patients who had moderate negative symptoms prior to neuroleptic withdrawal. These symptoms returned to pretreatment levels beginning with the second week of reinstituting neuroleptic medication. There were no significant correlations between changes in positive and negative

Table 14-1. SADS subscales at baseline and following 6-week treatment with typical neuroleptic drugs

Scales	N	Mean ± SD		P
		Baseline	6 Weeks	
SADS positive	61	3.7 ± 2.5	2.5 ± 2.1	.0001
SADS negative	61	4.3 ± 3.4	3.0 ± 2.4	.006
SADS negative disorganization	61	3.6 ± 3.7	1.7 ± 2.7	.0001
Blunted affect	85	1.4 ± 1.2	1.2 ± 1.1	.60

Note. SADS = Schedule for Affective Disorders and Schizophrenia.

symptoms during either period. Tandon et al. (1990b) also noted improvement in both positive and negative symptoms in schizophrenic patients after 4 weeks of neuroleptic treatment. They observed a highly significant correlation between the degree of improvement in positive and negative symptoms.

Consistent with this observed covariance of positive and negative symptoms, there is some evidence that neuroleptics are ineffective in patients with negative symptoms only. Overall and Rhodes (1982) found no evidence for a neuroleptic effect on negative symptoms in a reanalysis of data from 473 schizophrenic patients who had a withdrawn-disorganized profile on the BPRS (high on emotional withdrawal, motor retardation, blunted affect, and disorganization; low on hallucinations, unusual thought content, hostility, suspiciousness, anxiety, and excitement). These patients would perhaps be diagnosed as residual schizophrenia by DSM-III (American Psychiatric Association 1980) criteria.

Several studies have demonstrated an additive effect of a variety of psychosocial interventions and neuroleptic drugs on various dimensions of social function (Claghorn et al. 1974; Hogarty et al. 1974; Linn et al. 1979). These studies do not specifically delineate negative symptoms. The improvement in social function may have occurred without any change in negative symptoms, but this is unlikely.

DIPHENYLDIBUTYLPIPERIDINE NEUROLEPTIC DRUGS

The issue of a possible advantage of specific classes of neuroleptic drugs on negative symptoms has been raised by studies of both the diphenyldibutylpiperidine agents and the substituted benzamides. The diphenyldibutylpiperidines include, among others, pimozide, clopimozide, fluspirilene, and penfluridol.

In an 8-week double-blind trial of pimozide versus carpipramine, a tricyclic neuroleptic, patients with predominantly negative symptoms showed a nonsignificant trend for an advantage for pimozide (Kudo 1972). Lapierre and Lavallee (1975) reported that pimozide-treated patients were significantly less withdrawn and easier to communicate with and were more effectively involved in group therapy and more appropriate in their interpersonal relationships than fluphenazine-treated schizophrenic patients. Lapierre (1978) subsequently reported significantly greater improvement during 1 year of treatment with penfluridol compared to fluphenazine. However, no difference was noted between the two drug treatments at 8 weeks.

Fluspirilene was reported to be superior to fluphenazine decanoate on the social interest factor of the Nurses' Observation Scale for Inpatient Evaluation (NOSIE) (Honigfeld and Klett 1965) scale by Frangos et al. (1978). Pimozide, but not chlorpromazine, significantly reduced emotional withdrawal in chronic schizophrenic patients (Kolivakis et al. 1974). Emotional withdrawal was reported to be completely eliminated in 43% of the pimozide patients but none of the chlorpromazine patients. Haas and Beckmann (1982) reported that pimozide but not haloperidol produced significant improvement in affective blunting, emotional withdrawal, and anergia. Van Kammen et al. (1987) reported that pimozide improved the BPRS negative (withdrawal-retardation) during a 4-week treatment period in 12 schizophrenic patients. Changes in BPRS thought disorder and withdrawal-retardation scales were significantly correlated. Feinberg et al. (1988) reported that pimozide was effective in decreasing a wide range of negative symptoms over a 6-week period as measured by the PANSS in 10 treatment-resistant schizophrenic patients. As this study had no placebo or other neuroleptic group, the results are difficult to interpret.

Although these studies would appear to suggest that diphenyl-dibutylpiperidine drugs are more effective in the treatment of negative symptoms than other neuroleptics, caution is urged before accepting this conclusion because these studies were generally marked by inadequate measures to assess negative symptoms, small samples, and short duration of treatment.

SUBSTITUTED BENZAMIDE DRUGS

A number of studies suggest that sulpiride, a substituted benzamide neuroleptic, may be effective in decreasing apathy and withdrawal and in increasing social participation in patients with marked negative symptoms (Cassano et al. 1975; Elizur and Davidson 1975; Mielke et al. 1977; Toru et al. 1972). These results would not be confirmed by Edwards et al. (1980) in a 6-week double-blind trial comparing high-dose sulpiride (1,800 mg/day) and trifluoperazine (15–45 mg/day) in 38 chronic schizophrenic patients, using the BPRS negative symptoms subscale as an indicator. Alfredsson et al. (1985) compared the effect of a moderate dose of sulpiride (800 mg/day) or chlorpromazine (400 mg/day) in 50 schizophrenic patients on a double-blind basis. Sulpiride significantly decreased the rating of negative symptoms using the Comprehensive Psychiatric Rating Scale and NOSIE scales during the first 2 weeks of treatment. Chlorpromazine was active at 4 weeks.

CLOZAPINE AND RELATED DRUGS AND NEGATIVE SYMPTOMS

There is a now a strong body of evidence from controlled clinical trials that suggests that clozapine, an atypical neuroleptic, may be superior to typical neuroleptic drugs in treating negative symptoms as well as positive symptoms. Clozapine was reported to be superior to chlorpromazine in treating negative symptoms in a large multicenter trial of schizophrenic patients (Fischer-Cornelssen and Ferner 1976). Two other early studies showed a strong trend in that direction (Gelenberg and Doller 1979; Gerlach et al. 1974), but one showed equal effectiveness for clozapine and chlorpromazine (Guirgius et al. 1977).

In a multicenter trial, Claghorn et al. (1987) compared chlorpromazine and clozapine in 151 schizophrenic patients (DSM-III criteria), none of whom had been hospitalized for more than 6 months. The withdrawal-retardation subscale of the BPRS was used to rate negative symptoms. Clozapine was significantly more effective than chlorpromazine in reducing anergia ratings at weeks 1–3, 5, 6, and 8 as well as at the final week of treatment.

In a recently completed multicenter trial, Kane et al. (1988) studied the effect of clozapine versus chlorpromazine in nearly 300 treatment-resistant chronic schizophrenic patients. Schizophrenic patients with a history of failure to respond to at least three neuroleptics of two different classes over 5 years were included. These patients were then treated prospectively with haloperidol at doses up to 60 mg/day for 6 weeks. No effect of haloperidol on BPRS positive or negative symptoms was found. Those patients with no clinical improvement or who were intolerant to haloperidol were next randomly assigned to a 6-week trial with chlorpromazine or clozapine. The mean peak dose of clozapine was 600 mg/day and of chlorpromazine it was 1,200 mg/day. Significant advantages of clozapine over chlorpromazine in BPRS positive symptoms and decreasing BPRS withdrawal-retardation scores were noted from week 1 to 6 and weeks 2 to 6, respectively. An analysis of covariance showed that the improvement in negative symptoms at 6 weeks was still significant even after covarying the improvement in positive symptoms (Honigfeld et al., unpublished data). Nurses' ratings on the NOSIE scale indicated significant improvement in social competence, social interest, personal neatness, and retardation at week 2–6, with the social interest factor ratings showing the greatest improvement. Thus the effect of clozapine on negative symptoms was somewhat slow compared to the effect on positive symptoms. There was no significant difference in extrapyramidal symptoms between the two groups because of the use of benztropine with chlorpromazine. Side effects such as sedation or extrapyramidal symptoms did not account for the difference in the effect of the two drugs on negative symptoms.

Meltzer et al. (1989a, 1989b) administered clozapine on an open basis to 51 treatment-resistant chronic patients for a mean (±SD) of 10.3 ± 18.1 months (range, 6 weeks to 35 months). Thirteen of the patients dropped out. Of the 38 patients who continued on clozapine, 31 (81.6%) showed improvement in positive symptoms of at least 20% on the BPRS. Increased affective arousal and responsivity, increased intellectual content, spontaneous speech, social drive, interest in activities, and social independence were also noted. When data from those subjects who improved were examined separately, there was no difference in the percentage of improvement in positive and negative symptoms. Nevertheless, there were trends for the percentage of improvement in negative symptoms to exceed the percentage of improvement in SADS positive symptoms. The proportion of patients with improvement in positive or negative symptoms ± 20% of baseline also did not differ. Of interest is the fact that improvement in negative symptoms occurred in seven of eight patients with no improvement in positive symptoms. Since our treatment program included psychosocial treatments along with clozapine and there was no drug comparison group, such improvement cannot be solely attributed to clozapine.

We have recently updated this series. Sixty-one treatment-resistant schizophrenic patients treated with clozapine for 6 weeks or longer symptoms were rated with the SADS and the BPRS. SADS subscales were as follows: positive symptoms (severity of delusions and hallucinations); negative depressive symptoms (loss of interest, slow speech, slow body movement, and depressed appearance); and negative disorganization symptoms (inappropriate affect, loosening of associations, poverty of content, and incoherence). The BPRS positive and anergia subscales were also used. Baseline and 6-week ratings are given in Table 14-2.

Significant decreases were present in all subscales except for the BPRS negative subscale, for which there was only a weak trend. The greatest decrease in symptoms was noted in the SADS-C disorganization subscale. Improvement in positive symptoms was still significant after covarying out improvement in the other subscales individually. Improvement in the SADS-C negative depression and disorganization subscales was also significant after covarying out improvement in positive symptoms.

We have found that clozapine treatment for 6 to 9 months significantly improved Quality of Life scale (Heinrichs et al. 1984) ratings in 21 treatment-resistant schizophrenic patients (Meltzer et al. 1989b). This scale includes an intrapsychic foundation factor, which consists basically of a group of negative symptoms: sense of purpose, motivation, curiosity, anhedonia, aimless inactivity, empathy, and emotional interaction. Of the 21 patients, 6 were able to be employed in the private sector, 5 had volunteer jobs, and 2 returned to school. Only 10 of the 21 (47.6%) were unable to work or study. Lindstrom (1987) also found that clozapine treatment facilitated work function.

These results suggest that clozapine can ameliorate some negative symptoms, rapidly and independently of improvement in positive symptoms. The effect appears to be present in patients with acute exacerbations as well as patients who are treatment resistant. In the latter group, symptoms such as inappropriate affect, poverty of thought content, incoherence, and loose association (disorganization) and depressive-like negative symptoms (loss of interest, slowed speech, slowed body movement, and depressed appearance) may be more responsive than symptoms such as emotional withdrawal and blunted affect. Assuming that these are three subtypes of negative symptoms, it would appear that there is heterogeneity to negative symptoms and that a hierarchy exists as to which are most clozapine sensitive.

There is some evidence that other clozapine-like atypical antipsychotic drugs are also able to ameliorate negative symptoms. Fluperlapine, a clozapine-like morphanthridine compound, slightly but significantly decreased ratings of the Apathy Syndrome using the European based AMDP system (AMDP 1979) of assessment (Woggon et al. 1984). These changes were much smaller than the improve-

Table 14-2. SADS and BPRS subscales at baseline and following 6-week clozapine treatment

| | | Mean ± SD | | |
Scale or item	N	Baseline	6 Weeks	P
SADS positive	77	3.8 ± 2.4	1.9 ± 2.1	.0001
SADS negative	77	3.2 ± 3.7	2.4 ± 2.6	.03
SADS disorganization	77	3.3 ± 3.3	1.5 ± 2.2	.0001
BPRS positive	50	16.0 ± 5.5	11.5 ± 4.3	.0001
BPRS negative	50	9.5 ± 3.7	8.8 ± 3.9	.12

Note. SADS = Schedule for Affective Disorder and Schizophrenia. BPRS = Brief Psychiatric Rating Scale.

ment in positive symptom-based syndromes such as Hallucinations and Paranoia, but the study was only 3 weeks in duration.

Piquindone (RO22-1319) is a novel antipsychotic agent with atypical properties suggestive of clozapine (Davidson et al. 1983). In a placebo-controlled study, it was found to produce a greater decrease in negative symptoms during a 2-week trial (Cohen et al. 1987a).

We are currently studying the effect of melperone, a clozapine-like butyrophenone (Bjerkenstedt 1978), in 30 treatment-resistant schizophrenic patients. Melperone had a greater effect on negative symptoms than previous treatment with typical neuroleptic drugs in some patients (Meltzer et al., unpublished data). Thus available evidence suggests clozapine-like atypical antipsychotic drugs may be able to ameliorate negative symptoms more so than typical neuroleptic drugs. This may be due to their ability to increase dopamine release (Meltzer et al., in press).

EFFECT OF PROPRANOLOL ON NEGATIVE SYMPTOMS

There have been two studies on the effect of the beta-adrenergic blocker propranolol on negative symptoms. Sheppard (1979) reported that propranolol decreased anergia, lack of social interaction, and withdrawal in chronic schizophrenia. Subsequently, Eccleston et al. (1985) reported that propranolol had a significantly greater effect than thioridazine in decreasing positive and negative symptoms in a group of chronic schizophrenic patients with a mean duration of illness of 19 years. The dose of thioridazine in this study may have been inadequate.

EFFECT OF L-DOPA AND d-AMPHETAMINE ON NEGATIVE SYMPTOMS

There is an extensive uncontrolled literature suggesting that the two indirect dopamine agonists, L-dopa and *d*-amphetamine, are effective when administered together with neuroleptics in alleviating certain types of negative symptoms (Angrist et al. 1973; Calil et al. 1971; Garfinkel and Stancer 1976; Meltzer 1985; Yaryura-Tobias et al. 1970a, 1970b). There have also been four controlled studies of L-dopa in adult schizophrenic patients indicating a positive effect on negative symptoms (Alpert et al. 1978; Buchanan et al. 1975; Gerlach and Luhdorf 1975; Inanaga et al. 1975). Notably, there was infrequent exacerbation of positive symptoms following the administration of L-dopa to these patients. The possibility that some of the improvement in activity and rapport noted in these studies might be secondary to reduction in extrapyramidal symptoms cannot be excluded.

d-Amphetamine in doses of up to 50 mg/day, administered to 48 chronic schizophrenic patients, 35 of whom were receiving neuroleptics, produced significant improvement in 32 of the 48 patients (Cesarec and Nyman 1985). Nine of 17 patients who had marked negative symptoms showed improvement with d-amphetamine. The ability of L-dopa and d-amphetamine to improve negative symptoms may be additional evidence that these symptoms may be related to decreased dopaminergic activity. Van Kammen and Boronow (1988) administered d-amphetamine or placebo intravenously to 30 schizophrenic patients while on and off pimozide. There was significant decrease in the BPRS negative symptom cluster 30 to 45 minutes after the amphetamine infusion. The change in negative symptoms was independent of improvement in positive symptoms. The improvement in negative symptoms was not diminished by pimozide. Improvement in negative symptoms occurred as a result of pimozide treatment (van Kammen et al. 1987) and was correlated with the improvement in negative symptoms due to amphetamine.

OTHER APPROACHES TO THE PSYCHOPHARMACOLOGIC TREATMENT OF NEGATIVE SYMPTOMS

Anticholinergic drugs have been reported to have a mood-elevating, activating effect in schizophrenic patients, with (Fisch 1987; Jellinek 1977) or without (Smith 1980) concomitant neuroleptic treatment. Fisch (1987) proposed that the activating effect of trihexyphenidyl in schizophrenic patients could be the basis for its effectiveness in the treatment of negative symptoms. Tandon et al. (1988) studied the effect of the open addition of trihexyphenidyl, 5 mg bid, to five neuroleptic-treated schizophrenic patients who had predominantly negative symptoms. Improvement was noted in BPRS emotional withdrawal, depressed mood, motor retardation, and blunted affect as well as the affective flattening, avolition-apathy, and anhedonia subscale of the Scale for the Assessment of Negative Symptoms at 4 and 8 weeks of treatment.

Cole et al. (1961) reported that monoamine oxidase inhibitors decreased negative symptoms and increased motor activity in schizophrenic patients but with an accompanying increase in positive symptoms. Bucci (1987) added tranylcypromine to 15 neuroleptic-treated schizophrenic patients who had predominantly negative symptoms. Improvement in BPRS negative symptom items began after 4 weeks of treatment, with dramatic improvement noted by the end of 4 months in both negative symptoms and total BPRS. In a control group of 15 patients, no change in total BPRS or negative symptoms was noted for 4 months. Following the addition of tranylcypromine, there was a marked decrease in total BPRS and negative symptom subscale scores in these patients as well. Although these results need to be replicated in an additional study, they are promising. They are consistent with the hypothesis that reversal of a decrease in dopaminergic activity is important in treating negative symptoms.

Another class of agents that has been reported to be an effective treatment for negative symptoms are the benzodiazepines and triazobenzodiazepines. There is some uncontrolled evidence suggesting improvement in negative symptoms by estazolam and alprazolam (Csernansky et al. 1984; Lingjaerde 1982; Wolkowitz et al. 1986). For example, Wolkowitz et al. (1988) studied the effect of the addition of alprazolam in doses of 1.5 to 5.0 mg/day to 12 schizophrenic patients treated with fluphenazine and trihexyphenidyl. Duration of treatment varied due to differing rates of titration of alprazolam to "optimal" dosages but optimal dose was given for 4 weeks. There was a main effect of alprazolam. There was no effect of optimal dose of alprazolam on the BPRS negative symptom scale or the Abrams and Taylor Scale of Emotional Blunting (Abrams and Taylor 1978). However, the authors commented on the decrease in negative symptoms, which accompanied the overall improvement noted. The group data they report do not seem to support these conclusions.

There have been several evaluations of the effect of peptides on negative symptoms in schizophrenic patients. No effect of cholecystokinin (Albus et al. 1986; Peselow et al. 1987) was found.

The papaverine-type calcium-channel blocker verapamil was found to have no significant effect on negative symptoms (Grebb et al. 1986).

CONCLUSION

The preponderance of evidence from large controlled studies indicates that negative symptoms can respond to neuroleptic or clozapine treatment in at least a substantial subgroup of schizophrenic patients. However, the evidence suggests that the response of negative symptoms is generally slower and less satisfactory than the response to positive symptoms. Further studies are needed to assess the effect of typical neuroleptics and clozapine on negative symptoms utilizing standardized instruments specifically designed to rate negative symptoms and with attention to the possibility that there are discrete subtypes of negative symptoms.

Chapter 15

Conclusion: Is Integration Possible?

Rajiv Tandon, M.D.
John F. Greden, M.D.

Chapter 15

Conclusion: Is Integration Possible?

T he foregoing chapters summarize current viewpoints about clinical aspects, underlying pathophysiologies, and treatment approaches for negative symptoms in schizophrenia. Their diversity indicates the "richness" and importance of this construct. The same diversity points to confusion in the field and underscores the difficulty in integrating the various findings. Is it possible to formulate a framework that might accommodate these apparently disparate findings and hypotheses? In approaching this question, we assumed that all the concepts and mechanisms described in previous chapters have validity, but that they represent different perspectives of the same entity (or possibly two). We also made the following preliminary observations. First, negative symptoms constitute an integral element of schizophrenic psychopathology. They may also occur in other psychiatric conditions, however. Second, the evidence is convincing that a negative syndrome exists. Although many definitions of negative symptoms are currently employed and unanimity is absent, some elements are constant. No final determination can be made yet about the appropriateness of narrow versus broad definitions; it is possible that both may be appropriate in different contexts. Third, in a longitudinal context, negative symptoms probably exist even before the onset of positive symptomatology and may be evident in impaired premorbid functioning. They are present through the psychotic phase, when they may be obscured by the more florid positive symptoms. In a substantial number of patients, they may persist as residual or "deficit" symptoms long after positive symptoms subside. Fourth, negative symptoms, if viewed as a single construct, appear to change in the course of schizophrenia. Their severity fluctuates through the illness, with an increase in the psychotic phase. This increase in negative symptomatology may precede the appearance of delusions and hallucinations in the prepsychotic phase, persist through the psychotic phase, and decrease more slowly in the postpsychotic phase, appearing as postpsychotic "depressive" symptomatology. In this phase of the illness, negative symptoms probably covary with positive symptoms and appear to be "neuroleptic responsive."

If we consider these associations with premorbid personality, longitudinal course, treatment responsiveness, prognostic significance, and implicated pathophysiologic mechanisms, it appears that investigators may be describing two distinct "kinds" of negative symptoms: 1) the nonenduring, phasic, or treatment-responsive variety; and 2) the enduring, deficit, or treatment-nonresponsive variety (See Table 15-1).

Authors in this volume have characterized these different types in various ways: primary and secondary nonenduring versus enduring deficit (Carpenter et al., Chapter 1); phasic and associated with good outcome versus persistent and associated with poor outcome (Kay,

Table 15-1. Two types of negative symptoms

Parameter	Nonenduring, phasic, treatment-responsive	Enduring, deficit, treatment-nonresponsive
Terminology	Nonenduring Phasic Treatment-responsive Transitory State (psychotic phase)	Enduring Persistent Treatment-nonresponsive Deficit Trait
Phase when present	Psychotic phase, and also in the pre- and postpsychotic periods	Present throughout the illness, but most apparent in a stable period, such as premorbid or chronic residual phase
Premorbid adjustment	??	Poor
Prognostic implication	May have no association with outcome or may predict good resolution of current psychotic exacerbation	Associated with poor outcome
Family history	+	+ +
Association with positive symptoms	Covary with positive symptoms in psychotic phase	Unrelated to positive symptoms or jointly related to some "severity" factor

Table 15-1. Two types of negative symptoms — Continued

Parameter	Nonenduring, phasic, treatment-responsive	Enduring, deficit, treatment-nonresponsive
Postulated patho-physiologic process neuro-transmitters Dopamine	? Decreased in meso-cortical region	?? Decreased
Acetylcholine	Increased muscarinic activity	??
Norepinephrine	Increased	Decreased
Serotonin	?	? Decreased
Neuroendocrine findings	DST nonsuppression Increased GH response to TRH	Blunted GH response to apomorphine
Structural (cerebral atrophy, enlarged ventricles)	±	+ +
Polysomnography	Decreased REM latency	Decreased slow-wave sleep
Response to neuroleptics	+ +; related to their covariance with positive symptoms	Poor
Effective treatment approaches	Pharmacotherapy; treat-ment of positive symp-toms; supportive therapy	Social skills training and other rehabilitative tech-niques

Note. DST = dexamenthasone suppression test. GH = growth hormone. TRH = thyrotropin-releasing hormone. REM = rapid eye movement.

Chapter 2); and treatment responsive versus treatment nonresponsive (van Kammen et al., Chapter 7). Pogue-Geile and Keshavan (Chapter 3) alluded to this distinction when they discussed the syndromic versus subtype characterization of the negative symptom construct. Silk and Tandon (Chapter 4) discussed the various rating scales with reference to those that can assess change (state) versus those that imply immutability (trait).

This distinction is also implicit in the various postulated underlying mechanisms. Van Kammen et al. (Chapter 7) suggested that while increased noradrenergic activity may be associated with phasic (psychotic) negative symptoms, decreased noradrenergic activity may contribute to persistent (deficit) negative symptoms. We (Chapter 6) suggested that increased muscarinic cholinergic activity is involved in the production of phasic negative symptoms; its role in deficit symptoms is unclear. Although Berman and Weinberger (Chapter 5) did not specify the phase or type of negative symptom associated with dopamine deficiency, their allusion to the Pycock model of mesolimbic-mesocortical dopamine balance suggested that this mechanism is involved in the phasic (psychotic) variety, although it may be involved in the enduring (deficit) type as well. The structural-developmental mechanisms that were discussed (enlarged ventricles and cerebral atrophy) appear to relate to the persistent or deficit negative symptoms.

With regard to treatment, pharmacologic approaches seem best suited to the nonenduring, phasic negative symptoms; the deficit variety appear to be more responsive to rehabilitative strategies.

Most authors noted no difference in the symptomatic profile of these two putative negative symptom types, although neuropsychological impairment appears to be more closely related to the deficit type. Mukherjee et al. (Chapter 11) suggested that such differences in symptomatic description may exist, with attentional impairment, affective blunting, and alogia being associated with poor premorbid function and, as a corollary, with the deficit variety; and anhedonia-asociality and avolition-apathy being associated with the nonenduring variety, or being nondiscriminating. It should be emphasized that none of the other authors noted such differences. If such differences are noted in future studies, however, they would be of obvious importance.

Although the above integration is admittedly speculative, it is consistent with most findings in the negative symptom literature. If confirmed in future studies, it may explain a number of apparently inconsistent findings, integrate disparate concepts and mechanisms, and thereby reduce some of the present confusion in the field. We wish to emphasize that we view both phasic and enduring negative symptoms as an integral part of schizophrenic psychopathology, although the two may have different clinical and neurobiologic features (Tandon et al. 1990c).

Even if the distinction between nonenduring and deficit negative symptoms is valid, important questions remain:

1. Phenomenologically, how does one differentiate between them?
2. How do these varieties of negative symptoms relate to one another in terms of longitudinal course and underlying pathophysiology? For example, does the severity of phasic negative symptoms increase or protect against deficit negative symptoms? Or are the two

unrelated? Is there any relationship between their underlying pathophysiologic bases?

3. Even if a particular pathophysiologic mechanism is associated with one or the other type of negative symptoms, does it represent a pathophysiologically meaningful mechanism or an epiphenomenon?

4. What strategy or combination of strategies can investigators adopt to distinguish between them?

5. Enduring or deficit negative symptoms may comprise elements of premorbid dysfunction and post-psychotic deterioration. Do distinct mechanisms may underly these two components? (Dequardo et al. 1990).

Alternative models can be proposed to explain apparently discrepant findings and integrate the various concepts of negative symptoms that currently exist. In any event, it is clearly important to identify etiologically distinct categories of negative symptoms if these exist, and the current data suggest that they do. It could be argued that if the present literature refers to fundamentally different types of negative symptoms, only one of these varieties represents "the real negative symptom syndrome." Although the negative symptom construct clearly needs to be refined, it would probably be counterproductive to embrace a narrow and exclusive definition at this early stage.

Although there are no simple answers to the questions raised above, some general guidelines can be recommended to researchers in this field. When studying the association of negative symptoms with any clinical or neurobiologic parameter, the phase of assessment and the rating instrument employed to measure negative symptoms is clearly important. Ideally, any relationship should be studied in different phases of the illness to evaluate its trait and state components. Even in a particular phase of the illness, the temporal pattern of the relationship should be traced to permit assessment of pathophysiologic significance.

Current data suggest that the negative symptom construct serves as a useful organizing principle in schizophrenia. Precise delineation of the construct and its underlying pathophysiologic basis still is underway. Reasonably effective management strategies are available, although a better understanding of the phenomenon hopefully will aid in the development of more efficacious treatments. We have made a beginning. We now must look to future research to provide more definitive answers.

References

Abrams N, Taylor MA: A rating scale for emotional blunting. Am J Psychiatry 135:226–229, 1978

Ackerly SS, Benton AL: Report of a case of bilateral frontal lobe defect. Res Publ Assoc Res Nerv Ment Dis 27:479–504, 1947

Aggleton JP, Passingham RE: Syndrome produced by lesions of the amygdala in monkeys (Macaca mulatta). Journal of Comparative and Physiological Psychology 95:961–977, 1981

Alanen YO, Rakkolainen V, Rasimus R, et al: Developing a global psychotherapeutic approach to schizophrenia: results of a five-year follow-up. Yale J Biol Med 58:383–402, 1985

Albus M, von Gellhorn K, Munch V, et al: A double-blind study with ceruletide in chronic schizophrenic patients: biochemical and clinical results. Psychiatry Res 19:1–7, 1986

Alfredsson G, Harnryd C, Wiesel F-A: Effects of sulpiride and chlorpromazine on autistic and positive psychotic symptoms in schizophrenic patients: relationship to drug concentrations. Psychopharmacology 85:8–13, 1985

Alpert M, Friedhoff AJ, Marcos LR, et al: Paradoxical reaction to L-dopa in schizophrenic patients. Am J Psychiatry 135:1327–1332, 1978

Alphs L, Summerfelt A, Lann H, et al: The Negative Symptom Assessment: a new instrument to assess negative symptoms of schizophrenia. Psychopharmacol Bull 25:159–163, 1989

Altamura AC, Buccio M, Colombo G, et al: Combination therapy with haloperidol and orphenadrine in schizophrenia. L'Encephale 12:31–36, 1986

AMDP: AMDP, Arbeitsgemeinschaft fur methodik und dokumentation in der Psychiatrie (Hrsg): Das AMDP-System. Manual zur Dokumentation Psychiatrischen Befunde. Berlin, Springer, 1979

American Psychiatric Association: Diagnostic and Statistical Manual of Mental Disorders, 3rd Edition. Washington, DC, American Psychiatric Association, 1980

American Psychiatric Association: Diagnostic and Statistical Manual of Mental Disorders, 3rd Edition, Revised. Washington, DC, American Psychiatric Association, 1987

American Psychological Association: Standards for Educational and Psychological Tests. Washington, DC, American Psychological Association, 1974

Andreasen NC: Affective flattening and the criteria for schizophrenia. Am J Psychiatry 136:946–947, 1979

Andreasen NC: Negative symptoms in schizophrenia: definition and reliability. Arch Gen Psychiatry 39:784–788, 1982

Andreasen NC: Scale for the Assessment of Negative Symptoms (SANS). Iowa City, IA, University of Iowa, 1983

Andreasen NC: Scale for the Assessment of Positive Symptoms (SAPS). Iowa City, IA, University of Iowa, 1984

Andreasen NC: Positive vs. negative schizophrenia: a critical evaluation. Schizophr Bull 11:380–389, 1985

Andreasen NC, Olsen SA: Negative vs. positive schizophrenia: definition and validation. Arch Gen Psychiatry 39:789–794, 1982

Andreasen NC, Olsen SA, Dennert JW, et al: Ventricular enlargement in schizophrenia: relationship to positive and negative symptoms. Am J Psychiatry 139:297–302, 1982

Andreasen NC, Nasrallah HA, Dunn V, et al: Structural abnormalities in the frontal system in schizophrenia: a magnetic resonance imaging study. Arch Gen Psychiatry 43:136–144, 1986

Andreasen NC, Ehrhardt JC, Swayze VW, et al: Magnetic resonance imaging in schizophrenia: the pathophysiologic significance of structural abnormalities. Arch Gen Psychiatry 47:35–44, 1990a

Andreasen NC, Flaum M, Swayze VW, et al: Positive and negative symptoms in schizophrenia: a critical reappraisal. Arch Gen Psychiatry 47:615–621, 1990b

Angrist B, Santhanathan G, Gershon S: Behavioral effect of L-dopa in schizophrenic patients. Psychopharmacologia 31:1–12, 1973

Angrist B, Santhanathan G, Wilks S, et al: Amphetamine psychosis: behavioral and biochemical aspects. J Psychiatr Res 11:13–23, 1974

Angrist B, Rotrosen J, Gershon S: Differential effects of amphetamine and neuroleptics on negative vs. positive symptoms in schizophrenia. Psychopharmacology 72:17–19, 1980

Angst J: European long-term followup studies of schizophrenia. Schizophr Bull 14:501–513, 1988

Anisman H, Ritch M, Sklar S: Noradrenergic and dopaminergic interactions in escape behavior: analysis of uncontrollable stress effects. Psychopharmacology (Berlin) 74:263–268, 1981

Annett M: Left, Right, Hand and Brain: The Right Shift Theory. Hillsdale, NJ, Lawrence Erlbaum, 1985

Antelman SM, Caggiula AR: Norepinephrine-dopamine interactions and behavior. Science 195:646–653, 1977

Arieti S: Primitive habits in the preterminal stage of schizophrenia. J Nerv Ment Dis 102:367–385, 1945

Asberg M, Montgomery S, Perris C, et al: CPRS: The Comprehensive Psychopathology Rating Scale. Acta Psychiatr Scand 271:5–27, 1978

Aylward E, Walker E, Betes B: Intelligence in schizophrenia: meta-analysis of the research. Schizophr Bull 10:380–389, 1984

Baron M, Gruen R, Rainer JD, et al: Family study of schizophrenic and normal control probands: implications for the spectrum concept of schizophrenia. Am J Psychiatry 142:447–455, 1985

Bartko JJ, Carpenter WT: On the methods and theory of reliability. J Nerv Ment Dis 163:307–317, 1976

Baumgartner A, Graf K-J, Kurten I: Neuroendocrine differences among subtypes of schizophrenic disorder? Neuropsychobiology 11:174–177, 1986

Beani L, Bianchi C: Effect of amantidine on cerebral acetylcholine release and content in the guinea pig. Neuropharmacology 12:283–289, 1973

Beckmann H, Waldmeier P, Lauber J, et al: Phenylethylamine and monoamine metabolites in CSF of schizophrenics: effects of neuroleptic treatment. J Neural Transm 57:103–110, 1983

Berenbaum H, Oltmanns TF, Gottesman II: Formal thought disorder in schizophrenics and their twins. J Abnorm Psychol 94:3–16, 1985

Berenbaum H, Oltmanns TF, Gottesman II: A twin study perspective on positive and negative symptoms of schizophrenia, in Positive and Negative Symptoms in Psychosis: Description, Research, and Future Directions. Edited by Harvey PD, Walker E. Hillsdale, NJ, Lawrence Erlbaum, 1987, pp 50–67

Berger M, Fleckenstein P, Olbrich R, et al: REM latency and cholinergic

REM induction test in depressives, patients with other psychotic disorders, and normal controls, in Biological Psychiatry 1988. Edited by Saletu B. Stuttgart, George Thieme Vlg, 1988

Berman KF, Zec RF, Weinberger DR: Physiological dysfunction of dorsolateral prefrontal cortex in schizophrenia, II: role of neuroleptic treatment, attention, and mental effort. Arch Gen Psychiatry 43:126–135, 1986

Berman KF, Weinberger DR, Shelton RC, et al: A relationship between anatomical and physiological brain pathology in schizophrenia: lateral cerebral ventricular size predicts cortical blood flow. Am J Psychiatry 144:127–128, 1987

Berman KF, Illowsky BP, Weinberger DR: Physiological dysfunction of dorsolateral prefrontal cortex in schizophrenia, IV: further evidence for regional and behavioral specificity. Arch Gen Psychiatry 45:616–622, 1988

Berrios GE: Positive and negative symptoms and Jackson: a conceptual history. Arch Gen Psychiatry 42:95–97, 1985

Besson JAO, Corrigan FM, Cherryman GR, et al: Nuclear magnetic resonance brain imaging in chronic schizophrenia. Br J Psychiatry 150:161–163, 1987

Biehl H, Maurer K, Schubert C, et al: Prediction of outcome and utilisation of medical services in a prospective study of first onset schizophrenics. Eur Arch Psychiatry Neurol Sci 236:139–147, 1986

Bilder RM, Mukherjee S, Reider RO, et al: Symptomatic and neuropsychological components of defect states. Schizophr Bull 11:409–419, 1985

Bird ED, Spokes EG, Iversen LL: Brain norepinephrine and dopamine in schizophrenia. Science 204:93–94, 1979

Bishop JR, Golden CJ, MacInnes WD, et al: The BPRS in assessing symptom correlates of cerebral ventricular enlargement in acute and chronic schizophrenia. Psychiatry Res 9:225–231, 1983

Bitter I, Jaeger J, Agdeppa J, et al: Subjective symptoms: part of the negative syndrome of schizophrenia. Psychopharmacol Bull 25:180–185, 1989

Bjerkenstedt L, Harnryd C, Grimm V, et al: A double-blind comparison of melperone and thiothixene in psychotic women using a new rating scale, the CPRS. Arch Psychiatr Nervenkr 226:157–172, 1978

Bleuler E: Dementia Praecox or the Group of Schizophrenias. Translated by Zinkin J. New York, International Universities Press, 1950

Bleuler M: Endokrinologische Psychiatrie, in Grundlagen Forschung Zur Psychiatrie 11B. Edited by Gruhle KW, Jung R, Mayer-Gross W, et al. Berlin, Springer-Verlag, 1964

Bleuler M: A 23-year longitudinal study of 208 schizophrenics and impressions in regard to the nature of schizophrenia, in The Transmission of Schizophrenia. Edited by Rosenthal D, Kety SS. Elmsford, NY, Pergamon, 1968, pp 3–12

Bleuler M: The Schizophrenic Disorders: The Long Term Patient and Family Studies. Translated by Clemens SM. New Haven, CT, Yale University Press, 1978

Bleuler M: Schizophrenic deterioration. Br J Psychiatry 143:78–79, 1983

Blumer D, Benson DF: Personality changes with frontal and temporal lobe lesions, in Psychiatric Aspects of Neurologic Disease, Vol 1. Edited by Benson DF, Blumer D. New York, Grune & Stratton, 1975, pp 151–170

Bogerts B, Meertz E, Schonfeldt-Bausch R: Basal ganglia and limbic system pathology in schizophrenia. Arch Gen Psychiatry 42:784–791, 1985

Borson S, Lipton B, Nininger J, et al: Psychiatry and the nursing home. Am J Psychiatry 144:1412–1418, 1987

Bowers MB: Central dopamine turnover in schizophrenic syndromes. Arch Gen Psychiatry 31:50–54, 1974

Bowers MB, Rozitis A: Regional differences in homovanillic acid concentrations after acute and chronic administration of antipsychotic drugs. J Pharm Pharmacol 26:743–745, 1974

Bowers MB, Swigar ME, Jatlow PI, et al: Early neuroleptic response: clinical profiles and plasma catecholamine metabolites. J Clin Psychopharmacol 7:83–86, 1987

Brambilla F: Neuroendocrine function in schizophrenia. Acta Psychiatr Belg 80:421–435, 1980

Brambilla F, Guerrini A, Rovere C, et al: Growth hormone release in schizophrenia. Neuropsychobiology 1:267–275, 1975a

Brambilla F, Guerrini A, Guastalla A, et al: Neuroendocrine effects of haloperidol therapy in chronic schizophrenia. Psychopharmacology 44:17–22, 1975b

Brambilla F, Rovere C, Guastalla A, et al: Gonadotropin response to synthetic gonadotropin hormone-releasing hormone (GnRH) in chronic schizophrenia. Acta Psychiatr Scand 54:131–145, 1976

Braun AR, Barone P, Chase TN: Interaction of D1 and D2 dopamine receptors in the expression of dopamine agonist induced behaviors, in

Advances in Experimental Medicine and Biology. Edited by Breese GR, Creese I. New York, Plenum, 1986, pp 151–166

Breier A, Wolkowitz OM, Doran AR, et al: Neuroleptic responsivity of negative and positive symptoms in schizophrenia. Am J Psychiatry 144:1549–1555, 1987

Brenner H, Boker W, Hodel B, et al: Cognitive treatment of basic pervasive dysfunctions in schizophrenia, in Schizophrenia: Scientific Progress. Edited by Schulz SC, Tamminga CA. New York, Oxford University Press, 1989, pp 358–367

Brickner RM: An interpretation of frontal lobe function based upon the study of a case of partial bilateral frontal lobectomy. Res Publ Assoc Res Nerv Ment Dis 13:259–351, 1934

Brickner RM: The Intellectual Functions of the Frontal Lobes: Study Based Upon Observation of a Man After Partial Bilateral Frontal Lobectomy. New York, Macmillan, 1936

Bridge TP, Kleinman JE, Karoum F, et al: Postmortem central catecholamines and antemortem cognitive impairment in elderly schizophrenics and controls. Neuropsychobiology 14:57–61, 1985

British Journal of Psychiatry: Negative symptoms in schizophrenia. 155 (Suppl 7), 1989

Brown GW: Length of hospital stay and schizophrenia: a review of the statistical studies. Acta Psychiatrica et Neurologica Scandinavica 34:414–430, 1960

Brown GW, Birley JLT: Crisis and life changes at the onset of schizophrenia. J Health Soc Behav 9:203–224, 1968

Brown R, Colter N, Corsellis JAN, et al: Post-mortem evidence of structural brain changes in schizophrenia. Arch Gen Psychiatry 43:36–42, 1986

Brozowski TS, Brown RM, Rosvold HE, et al: Cognitive deficits caused by regional depletion of dopamine in prefrontal cortex of rhesus monkeys. Science 202:929–932, 1979

Bucci L: The negative symptoms of schizophrenia and the monoamine oxidase inhibitors. Psychopharmacology 91:104–108, 1987

Buchanan FH, Parton RV, Warren JW: Double-blind trial of L-dopa in chronic schizophrenia. Aust N Z J Psychiatry 9:269–271, 1975

Buchanan RW, Heinrichs DW: The Neurological Evaluation Scale (NES): a structured instrument for the assessment of neurological signs in schizophrenia. Psychiatry Res 27:335–350, 1989

Buchanan RW, Kirkpatrick B, Heinrichs DW, et al: Clinical correlates of the deficit syndrome schizophrenia. Am J Psychiatry (in press)

Buhrich N, Crow TJ, Johnstone EC, et al: Age disorientation in chronic schizophrenia is not associated with premorbid intellectual impairment or past physical treatment. Br J Psychiatry 152:466–469, 1988

Bunnell BN: Amygdaloid lesions and social dominance in the hooded rat. Psychon Sci 6:93–94, 1966

Bunnell BN, Sodetz FJ, Shalloway DI: Amygdaloid lesions and social behavior in the golden hamster. Physiol Behav 5:153–161, 1970

Bunney BS, DeRiemer S: Effect of clonidine on dopaminergic neuron activity in the substantia nigra: possible indirect mediation by noradrenergic regulation of the serotonergic raphi system. Adv Neurol 35:99–104, 1982

Bunney WE, Hamburg DA: Methods for reliable longitudinal observation of behavior. Arch Gen Psychiatry 9:280–294, 1963

Burt DR, Creese I, Snyder SH: Properties of 3H-haloperidol and 3H-dopamine binding in calf brain membranes. Mol Pharmacol 12:800–812, 1976

Calil HM, Yesavage JA, Hollister LE: Low dose levodopa in schizophrenia. Communications in Psychopharmacology 1:593–596, 1971

Cameron DE: Early schizophrenia. Am J Psychiatry 95:567–578, 1938

Campbell DT, Fiske DW: Convergent and discriminant validation by the multitrait-multimethod matrix. Psychol Bull 56:81–105, 1959

Cannon TD, Mednick SA: Two pathways to schizophrenia in children at risk, in Straight and Devious Pathways From Childhood to Adulthood. Edited by Robins L, Rutter ML. Cambridge, UK, Cambridge University Press, 1990

Cannon TD, Mednick SA, Parnas J: Antecedents of predominantly negative- and predominantly positive-symptom schizophrenia in a high-risk population. Arch Gen Psychiatry 47:622–632, 1990

Cannon-Spoor HE, Potkin SG, Wyatt RJ: Measurement of premorbid adjustment in chronic schizophrenia. Schizophr Bull 8:460–484, 1982

Carlsson A: Antipsychotic drugs, neurotransmitters and schizophrenia. Am J Psychiatry 135:164–173, 1978

Carlsson A: The current status of the dopamine hypothesis of schizophrenia. Neuropsychopharmacology 1:179–186, 1988

Carpenter WT: Clinical research methods applicable to the study of treatment effects in chronic schizophrenic patients, in Perspectives in Schizophrenic Research: Presentations and Sessions of the VA Advisory Conference on Chronic Schizophrenia, Harpers Ferry, WV, 1979. Edited by Baxter DF, Melnechuk T. New York, Raven, 1980, pp 297–311

Carpenter WT, Buchanan RW: Domains of psychopathology relevant to the study of etiology and treatment of schizophrenia, in Schizophrenia: Scientific Progress. Edited by Schulz SC, Tamminga CT. New York, Oxford University Press, 1989, pp 13–22

Carpenter WT, Kirkpatrick B: The heterogeneity of the long-term course of schizophrenia. Schizophr Bull 14:645–652, 1988

Carpenter WT, Stephens JH: Prognosis as the critical variable in classification of the functional psychoses. J Nerv Ment Dis 170:688–691, 1982

Carpenter WT, Strauss JS, Bartko JJ: A flexible system for the identification of schizophrenia: a report from the International Pilot Study of Schizophrenia. Science 182:1275–1278, 1973

Carpenter WT, Sacks MH, Strauss JS, et al: Evaluating signs and symptoms: comparison of structured interview and clinical approaches. Br J Psychiatry 128:397–403, 1976

Carpenter WT, Heinrichs DW, Hanlon TE: Methodologic standards for treatment outcome research in schizophrenia. Am J Psychiatry 138:465–471, 1981

Carpenter WT, Heinrichs DW, Alphs LD: Treatment of negative symptoms. Schizophr Bull 11:440–452, 1985

Carpenter WT, Heinrichs DW, Wagman AMI: Deficit and non-deficit forms of schizophrenia: the concept. Am J Psychiatry 145:578–583, 1988

Carroll BJ, Greden JF, Haskett RF, et al: Neurotransmitter studies of neuroendocrine pathology in depression. Acta Psychiatr Scand 61 (suppl 280):183–189, 1980

Casamenti F, Cosi C, Pepeu G: Effects of D_1 and D_2 dopamine agonists and antagonists on cortical acetylcholine release in vivo, in Cellular and Molecular Basis of Cholinergic Function. Edited by Dowdall MJ, Hawthorne JN. New York, VCH Publishers, 1987, pp 245–249

Casey JF, Lasky JJ, Klett CJ, et al: Treatment of schizophrenic reactions with phenothiazine derivatives: a comparative study of chlorpromazine, trifluoperazine, methazine, procloparazine, perphenazine, phenobarbital. Am J Psychiatry 117:97–105, 1960a

Casey JF, Bennett IF, Lindley C, et al: Drug therapy in schizophrenia: a controlled study of the relative effectiveness of chlorpromazine, promazine, phenobarbital and placebo. Arch Gen Psychiatry 2:210–220, 1960b

Cassano GB, Castrogiovanni P, Conti L: Sulpiride versus haloperidol in schizophrenia: a double-blind comparative trial. Current Therapeutic Research 17:189–201, 1975

Cazzullo CL: Biological and clinical studies on schizophrenia related to pharmacological treatment. Recent Advances in Biological Psychiatry 5:114–143, 1963

Cazullo CL, Vita A, Sacchetti M, et al: Brain morphology in schizophrenic disorder: prevalence and correlates of diffuse (cortical and subcortical) brain atrophy. Psychiatry Res 29:257–259, 1989

Cesarec Z, Nyman AK: Differential effects to amphetamine in schizophrenia. Acta Psychiatr Scand 71:523–528, 1985

Chang W-H, Chen TY, Lee C-F, et al: Plasma homovanillic acid levels and subtyping of schizophrenia. Psychiatry Res 23:239–244, 1988

Chapman LJ, Chapman JP: Psychosis proneness, in Controversies in Schizophrenia: Changes and Constancies. Edited by Alpert M. New York, Guilford, 1985, pp 157–174

Chozick BS: The behavioral effects of lesions of the septum: a review. Int J Neuroscience 26:197–217, 1985

Chugani HT, Phelps ME, Mazziotta JC: Positron emission tomography study of human brain functional development. Ann Neurol 22:487–497, 1987

Ciompi L: Catamnestic long-term study on the course of life and aging of schizophrenics. Schizophr Bull 6:606–618, 1980

Ciompi L: Schizophrenic deterioration. Br J Psychiatry 143:79–80, 1983

Claghorn JL, Johnson EE, Cook TH, et al: Group therapy and maintenance of schizophrenics. Arch Gen Psychiatry 31:361–365, 1974

Claghorn J, Honigfeld G, Abuzzahab FS, et al: The risks and benefits of clozapine versus chlorpromazine. J Clin Psychopharmacol 7:377–384, 1987

Clark NL, Ray TS, Ragland RD: Chlorpromazine in chronic schizophrenic women: rate of onset and rate of dissipation of drug effects. Psychosom Med 25:212–217, 1963

Cleghorn JM, Brown GM, Brown PJ, et al: Growth hormone response to graded doses of apomorphine HCl in schizophrenia. Biol Psychiatry 18:875–885, 1983a

Cleghorn JM, Brown GM, Brown PJ, et al: Longitudinal instability of hormone responses in schizophrenia. Prog Neuropsychopharmacol Biol Psychiatry 71:545, 1983b

Cohen LH, Thale T, Tissenbaum MJ: Acetylcholine treatment of schizophrenia. Archives of Neurology and Psychiatry 51:171–175, 1944

Cohen JD, Van Putten T, Marder S, et al: The efficacy of piquindone: a new atypical neuroleptic in the treatment of the positive and negative symptoms of schizophrenia. J Clin Psychopharmacol 7:324–329, 1987a

Cohen RM, Semple WE, Gross M, et al: Dysfunction in a prefrontal substrate of sustained attention in schizophrenia. Life Sci 40:2031–2039, 1987b

Coiro V, Marchesi C, DeFerri A, et al: Pirenzepine inhibits growth hormone, but not thyrotropin response to TRH in patients with endogenous depression. Psychoneuroendocrinology 12:313–317, 1987

Cole JO, Jones RT, Klermann GL: Drug therapy. Progress in Neurology and Psychiatry 16:539–574, 1961

Cole JO, Goldberg SC, Davis JM: Drugs in the treatment of psychosis, in Psychiatric Drugs. Edited by Solomon P. New York, Grune & Stratton, 1966, pp 153–180

Conrad AJ, Scheibel AB: Schizophrenia and the hippocampus. Schizophr Bull 13:577–588, 1987

Coppen A, Abou-Saleh M, Milln P, et al: DST in depression and other psychiatric illness. Br J Psychiatry 142:498–504, 1983

Cornblatt BA, Lenzenweger MF, Dworkin RH, et al: Positive and negative schizophrenic symptoms, attention, and information processing. Schizophr Bull 11:397–408, 1985

Coryell W: The use of laboratory tests in psychiatric diagnosis: the DST as an example. Psychiatr Dev 3:139–159, 1984

Costall B, Naylor RJ: Modification of amphetamine effects by intracerebrally administered anticholinergic agents. Life Sci 11:239–253, 1972

Craine JF: The retraining of frontal lobe dysfunction, in Cognitive Rehabilitation: Conceptualization and Intervention. Edited by Trexler LE. New York, Plenum, 1982, pp 239–262

Creese I, Burt DR, Snyder SH: Dopamine receptor binding predicts clinical and pharmacological potencies of antipsychotic drugs. Science 192:481–483, 1976

Crow TJ: Molecular pathology of schizophrenia: more than one disease process? Br Med J 280:66–68, 1980a

Crow TJ: Positive and negative schizophrenic symptoms and the role of dopamine. Br J Psychiatry 137:383–386, 1980b

Crow TJ: A re-evaluation of the viral hypothesis: is psychosis the result of retroviral integration at a site close to the cerebral dominance gene? Br J Psychiatry 145:243–253, 1984

Crow TJ: The two-syndrome concept: origins and current status. Schizophr Bull 11:471–486. 1985

Crow TJ, Johnstone EC: Schizophrenia: nature of the disease process and its biological correlates, in Handbook of Physiology: The Nervous System V. Edited by Mountcastle VB, Plum F. Bethesda, MD, American Physiological Society, 1986, pp 843–869

Crow TJ, Mitchell WS: Subjective age in chronic schizophrenia: evidence for a subgroup of patients with defective learning capacity? Br J Psychiatry 126:360–363, 1975

Crow TJ, Stevens M: Age disorientation in chronic schizophrenia: the nature of the cognitive deficit. Br J Psychiatry 133:137–142, 1978

Crow TJ, Baker HF, Cross AJ, et al: Monoamine mechanisms in chronic schizophrenia: postmortem neurochemical findings. Br J Psychiatry 134:249–256, 1979

Crow TJ, Corsellis JAN, Cross AJ, et al: The search for changes underlying the type II syndrome of schizophrenia, in Biological Psychiatry. Edited by Perris C, Struwe G, Jansson B. Amsterdam, Elsevier, 1981, pp 727–731

Crow TJ, Owens DGC, Johnstone EC, et al: Does tardive dyskinesia exist? Mod Probl Pharmacopsychiatry 21:206–219, 1983

Crow TJ, Ferrier JN, Johnstone EC: The two syndrome concept and neuroendocrinology of schizophrenia. Psychiatr Clin North Am 9:99–113, 1986

Crow TJ, Colter N, Brown R, et al: Lateralized asymmetry of temporal horn enlargement in schizophrenia. Schizophrenia Research 1:155–156, 1988

Crow TJ, DeLisi LE, Johnstone EC: Concordance by sex in sibling pairs with schizophrenia is paternally inherited: evidence for a pseudoautosomal locus. Br J Psychiatry 155:92–97, 1989a

Crow TJ, Colter N, Frith EC, et al: Developmental arrest of cerebral asymmetries in early onset schizophrenia. Psychiatry Res 29:247–253, 1989b

Csernansky JG, Lombrozo L, Gulevich GD, et al: Treatment of negative schizophrenic symptoms with alprazolam: a preliminary open-blind study. J Clin Psychopharmacol 6:349–352, 1984

Daniel DG, Weinberger DR, Breslin N, et al: The effect of dopamine agonists on CBF and negative symptoms in schizophrenia. Schizophrenia Research 3:28, 1990

Davidson AB, Boff I, MacNeil DA, et al: Pharmacological effects of D1022-1319, a new antipsychotic agent. Psychopharmacology 79:32–39, 1983

Davidson M, Davis KL: A comparison of plasma homovanillic acid concentration in schizophrenic patients and normal controls. Arch Gen Psychiatry 45:561–563, 1988

Davila R, Manero E, Zumarraga M, et al: Plasma homovanillic acid as a predictor of response to neuroleptics. Arch Gen Psychiatry 45:561–563, 1988

Davis BM, Davis KL, Mohs RC, et al: Evaluating prolactin response to dopamine agonists in schizophrenia: methodological problems. Arch Gen Psychiatry 42:259–264, 1985

Davis KL, Hollister LE, Berger PS, et al: Cholinergic imbalance hypothesis of psychoses and movement disorders: strategies for evaluation. Psychopharmacology Communications 1:533–543, 1975

Davis KL, Hollister LE, Overall J, et al: Physostigmine: effects on cognition and affect in normal subjects. Psychopharmacology 51:23–27, 1976

Davison K, Bagley CR: Schizophrenia-life psychoses associated with organic disorders of the central nervous system, in Current Problems in Neuropsychiatry: Schizophrenia, Epilepsy, the Temporal Lobe. Edited by Herrington R. Br J Psychiatry Special Publication No. 4: 113–184, 1969

Day R, Nielsen JA, Korlen A, et al: Stressful life events preceding the acute onset of schizophrenia: a cross-national study from the World Health Organisation. Cult Med Psychiatry 11:123–205, 1987

de Leon J, Simpson GM, Wilson WH: Comparison of negative symptom assessment scales. New Research, American Psychiatric Association annual meeting. San Francisco, CA, 1989, p 33

DeMilio L: TRH response pattern in adolescent schizophrenic males. Br J Psychiatry 145:649–651, 1984

Dequardo JR, Goldman R, Tandon R, et al: Ventricle-brain ratio, cognitive function, educational achievement, and premorbid function in schizophrenia. Biol Psychiatry 27:107A, 1990

Dickinson SL, Gadie B, Tulloch IF: Alpha-1 and alpha-2 adrenoreceptor antagonists differentially influence locomotor and stereotyped behavior induced by d-amphetamine and apomorphine in the rat. Psychopharmacology 96:512–527, 1988

Dicks D, Myers RE, Kling A: Uncus and amygdala lesions: effects on social behavior in the free-ranging rhesus monkey. Science 165:69–71, 1969

Dieterle DM, Albus MI, Eben E, et al: Preliminary results with the Munich version of the Andreasen scale: assessment of productive and negative symptoms in chronic schizophrenia patients. Pharmacopsychiatry 19:96–100, 1986

Dilsaver SC: Cholinergic mechanisms in depression. Brain Res Rev 11:285–316, 1986

Dinan TG, Aston-Jones G: Chronic haloperidol inactivates brain noradrenergic neurons. Brain Res 325:385–388, 1985

Doane JA, Falloon IR, Goldstein MJ, et al: Parental affective style and the treatment of schizophrenia: predicting course of illness and social functioning. Arch Gen Psychiatry 42:34–42, 1985

Docherty JP, van Kammen DP, Siris SG, et al: Stages of onset of schizophrenic psychosis. Am J Psychiatry 135:420–426, 1978

Domino EF, Olds ME: Cholinergic inhibition of self-stimulation behavior. Journal of Pharmacology 164:202–211, 1968

Donlon P, Blacker K: Stages of schizophrenic decompensation and reintegration. J Nerv Ment Dis 157:200–208, 1973

Donnelly EF, Weinberger DR, Waldman IN, et al: Cognitive impairment associated with morphological brain abnormalities on computed tomography in chronic schizophrenic patients. J Nerv Ment Dis 168:305–308, 1980

Douglass AB, Tandon R, Shipley JE: EEG sleep in schizophrenia and affective disorders. Biol Psychiatry 25:203a, 1989

Duvoisin RC: Cholinergic-anticholinergic antagonism in parkinsonism. Arch Neurol 17:124–136, 1967

Dworkin RH, Lenzenweger MF: Symptoms and the genetics of schizophrenia: implications for diagnosis. Am J Psychiatry 141:1541–1546, 1984

Dworkin RH, Saczynaki K: Individual differences in hedonic capacity. Journal of Personality Research 48:620–626, 1984

Dworkin RH, Lenzenweger MF, Moldin SO, et al: A multidimensional approach to the genetics of schizophrenia. Am J Psychiatry 145:1077–1083, 1988

Eccleston D, Fairbairn AF, Hassanayeh F, et al: The effect of propranolol and thioridazine on positive and negative symptoms of schizophrenia. Br J Psychiatry 147:623–630, 1985

Edwards JG, Alexander JR, Alexander MS, et al: Controlled trial of sulpiride in chronic schizophrenic patients. Br J Psychiatry 137:522–529, 1980

Elizur A, Davidson S: The evaluation of the anti-autistic activity of sulpiride. Current Therapeutic Research 18:578–584, 1975

Elsworth JD, Leahy DJ, Roth RH, et al: Homovanillic acid concentrations in brain, CSF, and plasma as indicators of central dopamine function in primates. J Neural Transm 68:51–62, 1987

Endicott J, Spitzer RL: The Schedule for Affective Disorders and Schizophrenia. Arch Gen Psychiatry 35:837–844, 1978

Falloon IR, Liberman RP: Interactions between drug and psychosocial therapy in schizophrenia. Schizophr Bull 9:543–554, 1983

Falloon IR, Pederson J: Family management in the prevention of morbidity of schizophrenia: the adjustment of the family unit. Br J Psychiatry 147:156–163, 1985

Falloon IR, Boyd JL, McGill CW, et al: Family management in the prevention of morbidity of schizophrenia: clinical outcome of a two-year longitudinal study. Arch Gen Psychiatry 42:887–896, 1985

Farde L, Wiesel F-A, Hall H, Halldin C, et al: No D2 receptor increase in PET study of schizophrenia. Arch Gen Psychiatry 44:671–672, 1987

Farde L, Wiesel F-A, Stone-Elander S, et al: D2 dopamine receptors in neuroleptic-naive schizophrenic patients. Arch Gen Psychiatry 47:213–219, 1990

Farley IJ, Price KS, McCullough E, et al: Norepinephrine in chronic paranoid schizophrenia: above-normal levels in limbic forebrain. Science 200:456–458, 1978

Farley IJ, Price KS, McCullough E, et al: Brain norepinephrine and dopamine in schizophrenia (letter). Science 204:94, 1979

Farmer AE, McGuffin P, Spitznagel EL: Heterogeneity in schizophrenia: a cluster-analytic approach. Psychiatry Res 8:1–12, 1983

Farmer AE, McGuffin P, Gottesman II: Twin concordance for DSM-III schizophrenia. Arch Gen Psychiatry 44:634–641, 1987

Farmery SM, Owen F, Poulter M, et al: Reduced high affinity cholecystokinin binding in hippocampus and frontal cortex of schizophrenic patients. Life Sci 36:473–477, 1985

Fayen M, Goldman MB, Moulthrop MA, et al: Differential memory function with dopaminergic versus anticholinergic treatment of drug-induced extrapyramidal symptoms. Am J Psychiatry 145:483–486, 1988

Feighner JP, Robins E, Guze SB, et al: Diagnostic criteria for use in psychiatric research. Arch Gen Psychiatry 26:57–63, 1972

Feinberg I: Schizophrenia: caused by a fault in programmed synaptic elimination during adolescence. J Psychiatr Res 17:319–334, 1983

Feinberg SS, Kay SR, Elijovich LR, et al: Pimozide treatment of the negative schizophrenic syndrome: an open trial. J Clin Psychiatry 49:235–238, 1988

Ferrier IN: Endocrinology and psychosis. Br Med J 43:672–688, 1987

Ferrier IN, Arendt J, Johnstone EC, et al: Reduced nocturnal melatonin secretions in chronic schizophrenia: relationships to body weight. Clin Endocrinol (Oxf) 17:181–187, 1982

Ferrier IN, Johnstone EC, Crow TJ, et al: Anterior pituitary hormone secretion in chronic schizophrenics: responses to administration of hypothalamic releasing hormones. Arch Gen Psychiatry 40:755–761, 1983a

Ferrier IN, Roberts GW, Crow TJ, et al: Reduced cholecystokinin-like and somatostatin-like immunoreactivity is associated with negative symptoms in schizophrenia. Life Sci 33:475–482, 1983b

Ferrier IN, Johnstone EC, Crow TJ: Hormonal effects of apomorphine in schizophrenia. Br J Psychiatry 144:349–357, 1984

Fisch RJ: Trihexiphenidyl abuse: therapeutic implications for negative symptoms of schizophrenia. Acta Psychiatr Scand 75:91–94, 1987

Fischer-Cornelssen KA, Ferner VJ: An example of European multicenter trials: multispectral analysis of clozapine. Psychopharmacol Bull 12:34–39, 1976

Fish B: Neurobiologic antecedents of schizophrenia in children: evidence for an inherited, congenital neurointegrative defect. Arch Gen Psychiatry 34:1297–1313, 1977

Folstein MF, Folstein SE, McHugh PR: Mini-Mental State: a practical method for grading the cognitive state of patients for the clinician. J Psychiatr Res 12:189–198, 1975

Fonberg E, Kostarczyk J: Motivational role of social reinforcement in dogman relations. Acta Neurobiol Exp (Warsaw) 40:117–136, 1980

Foote SL, Bloom FE, Aston-Jones G: Nucleus locus coeruleus: new evidence of anatomical and physiological specificity. Physiol Rev 63:844–914, 1983

Forrer GR, Miller JJ: Atropine coma: a somatic treatment in psychiatry. Am J Psychiatry 115:455–458, 1958

Frangos H, Zissis NP, Leontopoulos I, et al: Double-blind therapeutic evaluation of fluspirilene with fluphenazine decanoate in chronic schizophrenics. Acta Psychiatr Scand 57:436–446, 1978

Freedman R: Interactions of antipsychotic drugs with norepinephrine and cerebellar neuronal circuitry: implications for the psychobiology of psychosis. Biol Psychiatry 12:181–196, 1977

Friedberg J: Shock treatment, brain damage and memory loss: a neurological perspective. Am J Psychiatry 117:1113–1118, 1961

Friedhoff AJ: A dopamine dependent restitutive system for the maintainence of mental normalcy. Ann NY Acad Sci 463:47–52, 1986

Friedhoff AJ: Dopamine as a mediator of a central stabilizing system. Neuropsychopharmacology 1:189–191, 1988

Friedhoff AJ, Alpert M: A dopaminergic-cholinergic mechanism in production of psychotic symptoms. Biol Psychiatry 6:165–169, 1973

Fuster JM: The Prefrontal Cortex. New York, Raven, 1980

Ganguli R, Reynolds CF, Kupfer DJ: Electroencephalographic sleep in young never-medicated schizophrenics. Arch Gen Psychiatry 44:36–44, 1987

Garfinkel PE, Stancer HC: L-dopa and schizophrenia. Canadian Psychiatric Association Journal 21:27–29, 1976

Gattaz WF, Riederer P, Reynolds GP, et al: Dopamine and noradrenaline in the cerebrospinal fluid of schizophrenic patients. Psychiatry Res 8:243–250, 1983

Gelenberg AJ, Doller JC: Clozapine versus chlorpromazine for the treatment of schizophrenia: preliminary results from a double-blind study. J Clin Psychiatry 40:238–240, 1979

Gerlach J, Luhdorf K: The effect of L-dopa on young patients with simple schizophrenia, treated with neuroleptic drugs: a double-blind crossover trial with madopar and placebo. Psychopharmacologia (Berlin) 44:105–110, 1975

Gerlach J, Koppelhus P, Helweg E, et al: Clozapine and haloperidol in a single-blind cross-over trial:therapeutic and biochemical aspects in the treatment of schizophrenia. Acta Psychiatr Scand 50:410–424, 1974

Gershon ES, DeLisi LE, Hamovit J, et al: A controlled family study of chronic psychoses, schizophrenia and schizoaffective disorder. Arch Gen Psychiatry 45:328–336, 1988

Gershon S, Olariu J: A new psychotomimetic, its antagonism by tetrahydroaminoacrin and its comparison with LSD, mescaline, and sernyl. Journal of Neuropsychiatry 1:283–292, 1960

Geschwind N, Levitsky W: Left-right asymmetry in temporal speech region. Science 161:186–187, 1968

Gibbons RD, Lewine RRJ, Davis JM, et al: An empirical test of a Kraepelinian vs. a Bleulerian view of negative symptoms. Schizophr Bull 11:390–396, 1985

Gil-Ad I, Dickerman Z, Weizman R, et al: Abnormal growth hormone response to LRH and TRH in adolescent schizophrenic boys. Am J Psychiatry 138:357–360, 1981

Gjessing R, Gjessing L: Some main trends in the clinical aspects of periodic catatonia. Acta Psychiatr Scand 37:1–13, 1961

Glowinski J, Herve D, Tassin JP: Heterologous regulation of receptors on target cells of dopamine neurons in the prefrontal cortex, nucleus accumbens and striatum. Ann NY Acad Sci 137:112–123, 1988

Goetz KL, van Kammen DP: Computerized axial tomography scans and subtypes of schizophrenia. J Nerv Ment Dis 174:31–41, 1986

Goldberg SC: Negative and deficit symptoms in schizophrenia do respond to neuroleptics. Schizophr Bull 11:453–456, 1985

Goldberg SC, Klerman GL, Cole JO: Changes in schizophrenic psychopathology and ward behavior as a function of phenothiazine treatment. Br J Psychiatry 111:120–135, 1965

Goldberg SC, Schooler NR, Mattson N: Paranoid and withdrawal symptoms in schizophrenia: differential symptom reduction over time. J Nerv Ment Dis 145:158–162, 1967

Goldberg TE, Weinberger DR: Methodological issues in the neuropsychological approach to schizophrenia, in Handbook of Schizophrenia, Vol 1: The Neurology of Schizophrenia. Edited by Nasrallah HA, Weinberger DR. New York, Elsevier Science Publishers, 1986, pp 141–156

Gomes UCR, Shanley BC, Potgieter L, et al: Noradrenergic overactivity in chronic schizophrenia: evidence based on cerebrospinal fluid noradrenaline and cyclic nucleotide concentrations. Br J Psychiatry 137:346–351, 1980

Goodman R: Are complications of pregnancy and birth causes of schizophrenia? Dev Med Child Neurol 30:391–394, 1988

Gorham DR, Polorny AD: Effects of a phenothiazine and/or group psychotherapy with schizophrenics. Diseases of the Nervous System 25:77–86, 1964

Gottesman II: Severity/concordance and diagnostic refinement in the

Maudsley-Bethlem schizophrenic twin study, in The Transmission of Schizophrenia. Edited by Rosenthal K, Kety S. New York, Pergamon, 1968, pp 37–48

Gottesman II, Shields J: Schizophrenia and Genetics: A Twin Study Vantage Point. New York, Academic, 1972

Gottesman II, Shields J: Schizophrenia: The Epigenetic Puzzle. New York, Cambridge University Press, 1982

Grace AA, Bunney BS: Nigral dopamine neurons: intracellular recording and identification with L-dopa injection and histofluorescence. Science 210:654–656, 1980

Grant AD, Berg EA: A behavioral analysis of degree of reinforcement and ease of shifting to new responses in a Weigl-type card sorting problem. J Exp Psychology 38:404–411, 1948

Gray JA, McNaughton N: Comparison between the behavioral effects of septal and hippocampal lesions: a review. Neurosci Biobehav Rev 7:119–188, 1983

Grebb JA, Shelton RC, Taylor EH, et al: A negative double-blind, placebo-controlled clinical trial of verapamil in chronic schizophrenia. Biol Psychiatry 21:691–694, 1986

Greden JF, Tandon R, Haskett RF: Physostigmine-induced cholinergic excess: a proposed model for negative schizophrenic symptoms (Scientific Abstracts). San Juan, Puerto Rico, American College of Neuropharmacology, 1987

Green M, Walker E: Neuropsychological performance and positive and negative symptoms. J Abnorm Psychol 94:460–470, 1985

Green M, Walker E: Attentional performance in positive- and negative-symptom schizophrenia. J Nerv Ment Dis 174:208–213, 1986a

Green M, Walker E: Symptom correlates of vulnerability to backward masking in schizophrenia. Am J Psychiatry 143:181–186, 1986b

Grenhoff J, Svensson TH: Clonidine regularizes substantia nigra dopamine cell firing. Life Sci 42:2003–2009, 1988

Griesinger W: Mental Pathology and Therapeutics, 2nd Edition. Translated by Robertson CL, Rutherford J. New York, William Wood & Co, 1882

Guirgius E, Voinesko G, Gray J, et al: Clozapine (Leponex) vs chlorpromazine (Largactil) in acute schizophrenia: a double-blind controlled study. Current Therapeutic Research 21:707–719, 1977

Guy W: ECDEU Assessment Manual for Psychopharmacology, Revised

Edition. Washington, DC, U.S. Department of Health, Education, and Welfare, 1976

Haas S, Beckmann H: Pimozide versus haloperidol in acute schizophrenia: a double blind controlled study. Pharmacopsychiatry 15:70–74, 1982

Hamilton M: A rating scale for depression. J Neurol Neurosurg Psychiatry 23:56–62, 1960

Haracz JL: Neural plasticity in schizophrenia. Schizophr Bull 11:191–229, 1985

Harding CM: Course types in schizophrenia: an analysis of European and American studies. Schizophr Bull 14:633–643, 1988

Harris VJ: The dexamethasone suppression test and residual schizophrenia. Am J Psychiatry 142:659–660, 1985

Hartmann L, Roger M, Lemaitre BJ, et al: Plasma and urinary melatonin in male infants during the first 12 months of life. Clin Chim Acta 121:37–42, 1982

Haug JO: Pneumoencephalographic evidence of brain atrophy in acute and chronic schizophrenic patients. Acta Psychiatr Scand 66:374–383, 1982

Hebb DO: Man's frontal lobes: a critical review. Arch Neurol Psychiatry 54:10–24, 1945

Hecaen H, Albert ML: Disorders of mental functioning related to front lobe pathology, in Psychiatric Aspects of Neurologic Disease, Vol 1. Edited by Benson DF, Blumer D. New York, Grune & Stratton, 1975, pp 137–149

Hedlund JL, Vieweg BW: The Brief Psychiatric Rating Scale (BPRS): a comprehensive review. Journal of Operational Psychiatry 11:48–65, 1980

Heinrichs DW, Buchanan RW: Significance and meaning of neurological signs in schizophrenia. Am J Psychiatry 145:11–18, 1988

Heinrichs DW, Hanlon TE, Carpenter WT: The Quality of Life Scale: an instrument for rating the schizophrenic deficit syndrome. Schizophr Bull 10:388–398, 1984

Hemphill RE, Reiss M, Taylor AL: Study of histology of testis in schizophrenics and other mental disorders. Journal of Mental Science 90:681–695, 1944

Herz MI, Melville C: Relapse in schizophrenia. Am J Psychiatry 137:801–805, 1980

Hess EJ, Bracha HS, Kleinman JE, Creese I: Dopamine receptor subtype imbalance in schizophrenia. Life Sciences 40:1487–1497, 1987

Hiatt JF, Floyd TC, Katz PH, et al: Further evidence of abnormal non-rapid-eye-movement sleep in schizophrenia. Arch Gen Psychiatry 42:797–802, 1985

Hirsch SR: Depression 'revealed' in schizophrenia. Br J Psychiatry 140:421–424, 1982

Hobson JA, English JT: Self-induced water intoxication. Ann Intern Med 58:324–332, 1963

Hogarty GE: Expressed emotions and schizophrenic relapse, in Controversies in Schizophrenia. Edited by Alpert M. New York, Guilford, 1985, pp 354–365

Hogarty GE, Goldberg SC, Schooler NR, et al: Drugs and sociotherapy in the aftercare of schizophrenic patients. Arch Gen Psychiatry 31:603–618, 1974

Holsboer-Trachsler E, Buol C, Wiedemann K, et al: Dexamethasone suppression test in severe schizophrenic illness: effects of plasma dexamethasone and caffeine levels. Acta Psychiatr Scand 75:608–613, 1987

Honigfeld G, Klett J: The Nurses' Observation Scale for Inpatient Evaluation (NOSIE): a new scale for measuring improvement in chronic schizophrenia. J Clin Psychol 21:65–71, 1965

Honigfeld G, Gillis RD, Klett CJ: NOSIE-30: a treatment-sensitive ward behavior scale. Psychol Rep 19:180–182, 1966

Hornykiewicz O: Brain catecholamine in schizophrenia: a good case for noradrenaline. Nature 299:484–486, 1982

Hoskins RC, Pincus G: Sex hormone relationships in schizophrenic men. Psychosom Med 11:102–109, 1949

Huber G: Pneumencephalographische und psychopathologische Bilder bei endogen Psychosen. Berlin, Springer Verlag, 1957

Huber G, Gross G, Schuttler R, et al: Longitudinal studies of schizophrenic patients. Schizophr Bull 6:592–605, 1980

Huseman CA, Jugler JA, Schneider RG: Mechanism of dopaminergic suppression of gonadotrophin secretion in men. J Clin Endocrinol Metab 51:209–213, 1980

Huttenlocher PR: Synaptic density in human frontal cortex: developmental changes and effects of aging. Brain Res 163:195–205, 1979

Iager AC, Kirch DG, Wyatt RJ: A negative symptom rating scale. Psychiatry Res 16:27–36, 1985

Illowski BP, Kirch DG: Polydipsia and hyponatremia in psychiatric patients. Am J Psychiatry 145:675–683, 1988

Inanaga K, Inouee K, Tachibana H, et al: Effect of L-dopa in schizophrenia. Folia Psychiatrica et Neurologica Japonica 26:145–157, 1975

Ingvar DH, Franzen G: Abnormalities of cerebral blood flow distribution in patients with chronic schizophrenia. Acta Psychiatr Scand 50:425–462, 1974

Itil TM, Keskiner A, Holden JMC: The use of LSD and ditran in the treatment of therapy-resistant schizophrenics. Diseases of the Nervous System 30:93–103, 1969

Jackson JH: On temporary mental disorders after epileptic paroxysms. West Riding Lunatic Asylum Medical Report 5:105–129, 1875

Jackson JH: On postepileptic states: a contribution to the comparative study of insanities. Journal of Mental Science 34:490–500, 1889

Jacobi W, Winkler H: Encephalographische studien an chronisch schizophrenen. Archiv Psychiatr Nervenkr 81:299–332, 1927

Jacobsen B, Kinney DK: Perinatal complications in adopted and non-adopted schizophrenics and their controls: preliminary results. Acta Psychiatr Scand 62 (Suppl 285):337–346, 1980

Jacobson R: Disorders of facial recognition, social behaviour and affect after combined bilateral amygdalotomy and subcaudate tractotomy: a clinical and experimental study. Psychol Med 16:439–450, 1986

Jaeger J, Bitter I, Czobor P, et al: The measurement of subjective experience in schizophrenia: The Subjective Deficit Syndrome Scale. Compr Psychiatry 31:216–226, 1990

Jakob H, Beckmann H: Prenatal developmental disturbances in the limbic altocortex in schizophrenics. J Neural Transm 65:303–326, 1986

Janowsky DS, El-Yousef MK, Davis JM, et al: Antagonistic effects of physostigmine and methylphenidate in man. Am J Psychiatry 130:1370–1376, 1973

Jellinek T: Mood elevating effect of trihexiphenidyl and biperiden in individuals taking antipsychotic medication. Diseases of the Nervous System 38:353–355, 1977

Jellinek T, Gardos G, Cole JO: Adverse effects of antiparkinson drug withdrawal. Am J Psychiatry 138:1567–1571, 1981

Johnstone EC, Crow TJ, Frith CD, et al: Cerebral ventricular size and cognitive impairment in chronic schizophrenia. Lancet 2:924–926, 1976

Johnstone EC, Crow TJ, Mashiter K: Anterior pituitary hormone secretion in chronic schizophrenics: an approach to neurohumoral mechanisms. Psychol Med 7:223–228, 1977

Johnstone EC, Crow TJ, Frith CD, et al: The dementia of dementia praecox. Acta Psychiatr Scand 57:305–324, 1978a

Johnstone EC, Crow TJ, Frith CD, et al: Mechanism of the antipsychotic effect in the treatment of acute schizophrenia. Lancet 1:848–851, 1978b

Johnstone EC, Owens DGC, Gold A, et al: Institutionalism and the defects of schizophrenia. Br J Psychiatry 139:195–203, 1981

Johnstone EC, Crow TJ, Frith CD, et al: Adverse effects of anticholinergic medication in positive schizophrenic symptoms: theoretical and practical considerations. Psychol Med 13:513–527, 1983

Johnstone EC, Owens DGC, Frith CD, et al: The relative stability of positive and negative features in chronic schizophrenia. Br J Psychiatry 150:60–64, 1987

Johnstone EC, Frith CD, Crow TJ, et al: The Northwick Park "functional psychosis" study: diagnosis and treatment response. Lancet 2:119–125, 1988

Johnstone EC, Owens DGC, Bydder GM, et al: The spectrum of structural changes in the brain in schizophrenia: age of onset as a predictor of clinical and cognitive impairments and their cerebral correlates. Psychol Med 19:91–103, 1989

Jonason KR, Enloe LJ: Alterations in social behavior following septal and amygdaloid lesions in the rat. Journal of Comparative and Physiological Psychology 75:286–301, 1971

Kane J, Honigfeld G, Singer J, et al: Clozapine for the treatment-resistant schizophrenic. Arch Gen Psychiatry 45:789–796, 1988

Karoum F, Karson CN, Bigelow LB, et al: Preliminary evidence of reduced combined output of dopamine and its metabolites in chronic schizophrenia. Arch Gen Psychiatry 44:604–607, 1987

Kasper S, Moises HW, Beckmann H: The anticholinergic biperiden in depressive disorders. Pharmacopsychiatria 14:195–198, 1981

Kay SR: Positive and Negative Syndrome Scale (PANSS) training film. Piscataway, NJ, Janssen Research Foundation, 1988

Kay SR, Lindenmayer JP: Outcome predictors in acute schizophrenia: prospective significance of background and clinical dimensions. J Nerv Ment Dis 175:152–160, 1987

Kay SR, Murrill LM: Predicting outcome of schizophrenia: significance of symptom profiles and outcome dimensions. Compr Psychiatry 31:91–102, 1990

Kay SR, Opler LA: The positive-negative dimension in schizophrenia: its validity and significance. Psychiatr Dev 5:79–103, 1987

Kay SR, Singh MM: The positive-negative distinction in drug-free schizophrenic patients: stability, response to neuroleptics, and prognostic significance. Arch Gen Psychiatry 46:711–718, 1989

Kay SR, Fiszbein A, Opler LA: Negative symptoms rating scale: limitations in psychometric and research methodology. Psychiatry Res 19:169–170, 1986a

Kay SR, Fiszbein A, Lindenmayer JP, et al: Positive and negative syndromes in schizophrenia as a function of chronicity. Acta Psychiatr Scand 74:507–518, 1986b

Kay SR, Opler LA, Fiszbein A: Significance of positive and negative syndromes in chronic schizophrenia. Br J Psychiatry 149:439–448, 1986c

Kay SR, Fiszbein A, Opler LA: The Positive and Negative Syndrome Scale (PANSS) for schizophrenia. Schizophr Bull 13:261–276, 1987a

Kay SR, Opler LA, Fiszbein A: Positive and Negative Syndrome Scale (PANSS) Rating Manual. San Rafael, CA, Social and Behavioral Sciences Documents, 1987b

Kay SR, Opler LA, Lindenmayer JP: Reliability and validity of the Positive and Negative Syndrome Scale for schizophrenics. Psychiatry Res 23:99–110, 1988

Kay SR, Opler LA, Lindenmayer JP: The Positive and Negative Syndrome Scale (PANSS): rationale and standardization. Br J Psychiatry 155 (Suppl 7):59–65, 1989

Keefe RSE, Mohs RC, Losonczy MF, et al: Premorbid sociosexual functioning and longterm outcome in schizophrenia. Am J Psychiatry 146:206–211, 1989

Keilp JG, Sweeney JA, Jacobsen P, et al: Cognitive impairment in schizophrenia: specific relations to ventricular size and negative symptomatology. Biol Psychiatry 24:47–55, 1988

Kemali D, Delvecchio M, Maj M: Increased noradrenaline levels in CSF and plasma of schizophrenic patients. Biol Psychiatry 17:711–717, 1982

Kemali D, Maj M, Galderisi S, et al: Clinical and neuropsychological correlates of cerebral ventricular enlargement in schizophrenia. J Psychiatr Res 19:587–596, 1985

Kemali D, Maj M, Galderisi S, Salvati A, et al: Clinical, biological, and neuropsychological features associated with lateral ventricular enlargement in DSM-III schizophrenic disorder. Psychiatry Res 21:137–149, 1987

Kendler KS: Diagnostic approaches to schizotypal personality disorder: a historical perspective. Schizophr Bull 11:538–553, 1985

Kendler KS, Davis KL: The genetics and biochemistry of paranoid schizophrenia and other paranoid psychoses. Schizophr Bull 7:689–709, 1981

Kendler KS, Hays P: Schizophrenia subdivided by the family history of affective disorder. Arch Gen Psychiatry 40:951–955, 1983

Kendler KS, Tsuang MT: Outcome and familial psychopathology in schizophrenia. Arch Gen Psychiatry 45:338–346, 1988

Kendler KS, Gruenberg AM, Tsuang MT: Psychiatric illness in first-degree relatives of schizophrenics and surgical control patients: a family study using DSM III criteria. Arch Gen Psychiatry 42:770–779, 1985

Keshavan M, Toone BK, Marshall W, et al: Neuroendocrine dysfunction in schizophrenia: a familial perspective. Psychiatry Res 23:345–348, 1988

Keshavan MS, Brar J, Ganguli R, et al: Dexamethasone nonsuppression and CT scan changes in schizophrenia. Biol Psychiatry 25:39A, 1989a

Keshavan MS, Brar J, Campbell K, et al: Growth hormone response to TRH and negative symptoms in schizophrenia. Biol Psychiatry 25:173–174A, 1989b

Keshavan MS, Reynolds C, Brar J, et al: Pretreatment sleep EEG parameters and prediction of response to haloperidol in schizophrenia. Biol Psychiatry 25:182A, 1989c

Kety SS: The significance of genetic factors in the etiology of schizophrenia: results from the national study of adoptees in Denmark. J Psychiatr Res 21:423–429, 1987

Kety SS, Rosenthal D, Wender PH, et al: The biologic and adoptive families of adopted individuals who became schizophrenic: prevalence of mental illness and other characteristics, in The Nature of Schizophrenia: New Approaches to Research and Treatment. Edited by Wynne LC, Cromwell RL, Matthysse S. New York, John Wiley, 1978, pp 25–37

Kirch DG, Weinberger DR: Anatomical neuropathology in schizophrenia: post-mortem findings, in Handbook of Schizophrenia, Vol 1: The

Neurology of Schizophrenia. Edited by Nasrallah HA, Weinberger DR. New York, Elsevier Science Publishers, 1986, pp 325–348

Kirch DG, Bigelow LB, Weinberger DR, et al: Polydipsia and chronic hyponatremia in schizophrenic inpatients. J Clin Psychiatry 46:179–181, 1985

Kirkpatrick B, Buchanan RW, McKenney P, et al: The Schedule for the Deficit Syndrome: an instrument for research in schizophrenia. Psychiatry Res 30:119–123, 1989

Kirkpatrick B, Buchanan RW: Anhedonia and the deficit syndrome of schizophrenia. Psychiatry Res 31:25–30, 1990

Klein DF: Importance of psychiatric diagnosis in prediction of clinical drug effect. Arch Gen Psychiatry 16:118–126, 1967

Kleinman JE, Weinberger DR, Rogol A, et al: Plasma prolactin concentrations and psychopathology in chronic schizophrenia. Arch Gen Psychiatry 39:655–657, 1982

Kleinman JE, Casanova MF, Jaskiw GE: The neuropathology of schizophrenia. Schizophrenia Bull 14:209–216, 1988

Kling A: Effects of amygdalectomy on social-affective behavior in non-human primates, in The Neurobiology of the Amygdala. Edited by Eleftheriou BE. New York, Plenum, 1972, pp 511–536

Kling A, Steklis HD: A neural substrate for affiliative behavior in nonhuman primates. Brain Behav Evol 13:216–238, 1976

Kling AS, Kurtz N, Tachiki K, et al: CT scans in subgroups of chronic schizophrenics. J Psychiatr Res 17:375–384, 1983

Knights A, Okasha MS, Salih MA, et al: Depressive and extrapyramidal symptoms and clinical effects. Br J Psychiatry 135:515–523, 1979

Kolakowska T, Gelder M, Fraser S: Plasma growth hormone and prolactin response to apomorphine. Br J Psychiatry 139:408–412, 1981

Kolakowska T, Williams AO, Adern M, et al: Schizophrenia with good and poor outcome, I: early clinical features, response to neuroleptics and signs of organic dysfunction. Br J Psychiatry 146:229–239, 1985

Kolivakis T, Azian H, Kingstone E: A double-blind comparison of pimozide and chlorpromazine in the maintenance of chronic schizophrenic patients. Current Therapeutic Research 16:998–1004, 1974

Kovelman JA, Scheibel AB: A neurohistological correlate of schizophrenia. Biol Psychiatry 19:1601–1621, 1984

Kraepelin E: Dementia Praecox and Paraphrenia. Edited by Barclay RB. Edinburgh, Livingston, 1919

Krawiecka M, Goldberg D, Vaughan M: A standardised psychiatric assessment for rating chronic psychiatric patients. Acta Psychiatr Scand 55:299–308, 1977

Kudo H: A double-blind comparison of pimozide with carpipramine in schizophrenic patients. Acta Psychiatr Belg 72:685–697, 1972

Kulhara P, Chadda R: A study of negative symptoms in schizophrenia and depression. Compr Psychiatry 28:229–235, 1987

Kulhara P, Kota SK, Joseph S: Positive and negative subtypes of schizophrenia: a study from India. Acta Psychiatr Scand 74:353–359, 1986

Kupfer DJ, Frank E, Jarrett DB, et al: The interrelationship of EEG sleep chronobiology and depression, in Biological Rhythms and Mental Disorders. Edited by Kupfer DJ, Barchas JD. New York, Guilford, 1989

Kurland AA, Hanlon TE, Tatom MH, et al: The comparative effectiveness of six phenothiazine compounds, phenobarbital, and inert placebo in the treatment of acutely ill patients: global measures of severity of illness. J Nerv Ment Dis 133:1–18, 1961

Lake CR, Sternberg DE, van Kammen DP, et al: Schizophrenia: elevated cerebrospinal fluid norepinephrine. Science 207:331–333, 1980

Lal S: Growth hormone and schizophrenia, in Psychopharmacology: The Third Generation of Progress. Edited by Meltzer HY. New York, Raven, 1987, pp 809–819

Lal S, Tolis G, Martin JB, et al: Effect of clonidine on growth hormone, prolactin, luteinizing hormone, follicle stimulating hormone, and thyroid stimulating hormone. J Clin Endocrinol Metab 41:827–832, 1975

Lal S, Nair NPV, Thavundayal JX, et al: Clonidine induced growth hormone secretion in chronic schizophrenia. Acta Psychiatr Scand 68:82–88, 1983

Langer G, Resch R, Keshavan MS, et al: TSH response to TRH stimulation may indicate therapeutic mechanisms of antidepressants and neuroleptic drugs. Neuropsychobiology 11:213–218, 1984

Langer G, Koinig G, Hafzinger R, et al: Response of thyrotropin to thyrotropin releasing as predictor of treatment outcome. Arch Gen Psychiatry 43:861–868, 1986

Lapierre YD: A controlled study of penfluridol in the treatment of chronic schizophrenia. Am J Psychiatry 135:956–959, 1978

Lapierre YD, Lavallee J: Pimozide and the social behaviors of schizophrenics. Current Therapeutic Research 18:181–188, 1975

Lawson WB, Waldman IN, Weinberger DR: Schizophrenic dementia: clinical and computed axial tomography correlates. J Nerv Ment Dis 176:207–212, 1988

Leff JP: A model of schizophrenic vulnerability to environmental factors, in Search for the Causes of Schizophrenia. Edited by Hafner H, Gatlar WF, Janzarik W. Berlin, Springer, 1987

Leff JP, Vaughn C: Expressed Emotions in Families. New York, Guilford, 1985

Leff JP, Hirsch SR, Gaind R, et al: Life events and maintenance therapy in schizophrenic relapse. Br J Psychiatry 123:659–660, 1973

Lenzenweger MF, Dworkin RH, Wethington E: Models of positive and negative symptoms in schizophrenia: an empirical evaluation of latent structures. J Abnorm Psychol 98:62–70, 1989

Leonard CM, Rolls ET, Wilson FAW, et al: Neurons in the amygdala of the monkey with responses selective for faces. Behav Brain Res 15:159–176, 1985

Levin S: Frontal lobe dysfunctions in schizophrenia, II: impairments of psychological and brain functions. J Psychiatr Res 18:57–72, 1984

Lewine RRJ: Negative symptoms in schizophrenia: editor's introduction. Schizophr Bull 11:361–363, 1985

Lewine RRJ, Sommers AA: Clinical definition of negative symptoms as a reflection of theory and methodology, in Controversies in Schizophrenia, Changes and Constancies. Edited by Alpert M. New York, Guilford, 1985, pp 267–279

Lewine RRJ, Fogg L, Meltzer HY: Assessment of negative and positive symptoms in schizophrenia. Schizophr Bull 9:368–376, 1983

Lewis SW: Congenital risk factors for schizophrenia (editorial). Psychol Med 19:5–13, 1989

Lewis SW, Reveley AM, Reveley MA, et al: The familial-sporadic distinction as a strategy in schizophrenia research. Br J Psychiatry 151:306–313, 1987

Lewis SW, Murray RM, Owen M: Obstetric complications in schizophrenia: methodology and mechanisms, in Schizophrenia: Scientific Progress. Edited by Schulz SC, Tamminga CA. New York, Oxford University Press, 1989, pp 56–68

Liberman RP, Evans CC: Behavioral rehabilitation for chronic mental patients. J Clin Psychopharmacol 5:8S–15S, 1985

Liberman RP, Mueser KT: Schizophrenia: psychosocial treatment, in Comprehensive Textbook of Psychiatry, Vol 5. Edited by Kaplan HI, Sadock BJ. Baltimore, MD, William & Wilkins, 1989, pp 792–805

Liberman RP, Massell HK, Mosk M, et al: Social skills training for chronic mental patients. Hosp Community Psychiatry 36:396–403, 1985

Liddle PF: The symptoms of chronic schizophrenia: a re-examination of the positive-negative symptom dichotomy. Br J Psychiatry 151:145–151, 1987a

Liddle PF: Schizophrenic syndromes, cognitive performance and neurological dysfunction. Psychol Med 17:49–57, 1987b

Liddle PF, Barnes TR: The subjective experience of deficits in schizophrenia. Compr Psychiatry 29:157–164, 1988

Liddle PF, Barnes TRE, Morris D, et al: Three syndromes in chronic schizophrenia. Br J Psychiatry 155 (Suppl 7):119–122, 1989

Liddle P, Crow TJ: Age disorientation in chronic schizophrenia is associated with global intellectual impairment. Br J Psychiatry 144:193–199, 1984

Lieberman JA, Kane JM, Sarantakos S, et al: Prediction of relapse in schizophrenia. Arch Gen Psychiatry 44:597–603, 1987

Lindberg D: A controlled study of 5 years' treatment with psychotherapy in combination with depot neuroleptics in schizophrenia, II: personality changes measured by ten selected Rorschach variables. Acta Psychiatr Scand (Suppl) 289:56–66, 1981

Lindenmayer JP, Kay SR, Opler LA: Positive and negative subtypes in acute schizophrenia. Compr Psychiatry 25:454–464, 1984

Lindenmayer JP, Kay SR, Friedman C: Negative and positive schizophrenic syndromes after the acute phase: a prospective follow-up. Compr Psychiatry 27:276–286, 1986

Lindstrom LH: Low HVA and normal 5HIAA CSF levels in drug-free schizophrenic patients compared to healthy volunteers: correlations to symptomology and family history. Psychiatry Res 14:265–273, 1985

Lindstrom LH: The effect of long-term treatment with clozapine in schizophrenia: a retrospective study in 96 patients treated with clozapine for up to 13 years. Acta Psychiatr Scand 76:524–529, 1987

Lingjaerde O: Effect of the benzodiazepine derivative estazolam in patients with auditory hallucinations: a multicenter double-blind, cross-over study. Acta Psychiatr Scand 65:339–354, 1982

Linn MW, Caffey FM, Klett J: Day treatment and psychotropic drugs in the aftercare of schizophrenic patients. Arch Gen Psychiatry 36:1055–1066, 1979

Linnoila M, Ninan PT, Scheinin M, et al: Reliability of norepinephrine and major monoamine metabolite measurements in CSF of schizophrenic patients. Arch Gen Psychiatry 40:1290–1294, 1983

Lohr JB, Jeste DV: Locus coeruleus morphometry in aging and schizophrenia. Acta Psychiatr Scand 77:689–697, 1988

Loosen PT: The TRH induced TSH response in psychiatric patients: a possible neuroendocrine marker. Psychoneuroendocrinology 3:237–260, 1985

Lorr M, Jenkins RL, Holsopple JQ: Multidimensional Scale for Rating Psychiatric Patients. Veterans Administration Technical Bulletin 10–507, 1953, pp 1–44

Lorr M, McNair DM, Klett CJ, et al: A confirmation of nine postulated psychotic syndromes. Am Psychol 15:495, 1960

Losonczy MF, Song IS, Mohs RC, et al: Correlates of lateral ventricular size in chronic schizophrenia, I: behavioral and treatment response measures. Am J Psychiatry 143:976–981, 1986a

Losonczy MF, Song IS, Mohs RC, et al: Correlates of lateral ventricular size in chronic schizophrenia, II: biological measures. Am J Psychiatry 143:1113–1118, 1986b

Luchins DJ, Lewine RRJ, Meltzer HY: Lateral ventricular size, psychopathology, and medication response in the psychoses. Biol Psychiatry 19:29–44, 1984

Luria AR: The frontal lobes and the regulation of behavior, in Psychophysiology of the Frontal Lobes. Edited by Pribram K, Luria AR. New York, Academic, 1973, pp 3–26

Luria AR: The Working Brain. New York, Basic Books, 1974

Mackay AVP: Positive and negative schizophrenic symptoms and the role of dopamine. Br J Psychiatry 137:380–383, 1980

MacMillan JF, Crow TJ, Johnson AL, et al: Expressed emotions and relapse in first episodes of schizophrenia. Br J Psychiatry 151:320–323, 1987

Malas KL, van Kammen DP, de Fraites EA, et al: Reduced growth hormone response to apomorphine in schizophrenic patients with poor premorbid social functioning. J Neural Transm 69:319–324, 1987

Malm U, May PRA, Dencker SJ: Evaluation of the quality of life of the schizophrenic outpatient: a checklist. Schizophr Bull 7:477–487, 1981

Mandel MR, Severe JB, Schooler NR, et al: Development and prediction of postpsychotic depression in neuroleptic-treated schizophrenics. Arch Gen Psychiatry 39:197–203, 1982

Manos N, Gkiouzepas J, Tzotzoras T, et al: Gradual withdrawal of antiparkinson medication in chronic schizophrenics: any better than the abrupt? J Nerv Ment Dis 169:659–661, 1981

Marder SP, van Kammen DP, Bunney WE: Prediction drug-free improvement from schizophrenic psychosis. Arch Gen Psychiatry 36:1030–1085, 1979

Mass R, Kling A: Social behavior in stump-tailed macaques (Macaca speciosa) after lesions of the dorsolateral frontal cortex. Primates 16:239–252, 1975

Mathai PJ, Chaturvedi SK, Michael A, et al: Evaluation of the reliability of the Scale for the Assessment of Negative Symptoms. Journal of Psychological Research 28:148–153, 1986

Mathew RJ, Partain CL, Prakash R, et al: A study of the septum pellucidum and corpus callosum in schizophrenia with MR imaging. Acta Psychiatr Scand 72:414–421, 1985

May HJ, Gazda GM, Powell M, et al: Life skill training: psychoeducational training as mental health treatment. J Clin Psychol 41:359–367, 1985

Mazzara C, Tandon R, Hariharan M, et al: DST in schizophrenic patients before and during neuroleptic treatment: association with symptomatology and ventricular size. Biol Psychiatry 25:41–42A, 1989

McDermott A, Conley R: Rehabilitation of the newly responsive schizophrenic (abstracts). Phoenix, AZ, American Occupational Therapy Association Meeting, 1986

McGlashan TH: A selective review of recent North American long-term followup studies of schizophrenia. Schizophr Bull 14: 515–542, 1988

McGlashan TH, Carpenter WT: Postpsychotic depression in schizophrenia. Arch Gen Psychiatry 33:231–239, 1976

McGlashan TH, Carpenter WT: Long-term followup studies of schizophrenia. Schizophr Bull 14:497–500, 1988

McGue M, Gottesman II, Rao DC: Resolving genetic models of the transmission of schizophrenia. Genet Epidemiol 2:99–110, 1985

McGuffin P, Farmer AE, Gottesman II, et al: Twin concordance for operationally defined schizophrenia: confirmation of familiality and heritability. Arch Gen Psychiatry 41:541–545, 1984

McGuffin P, Farmer A, Gottesman II: Is there really a split in schizophrenia: the genetic evidence. Br J Psychiatry 150:581–592, 1987

McKenna PJ, Kane JM, Parrish K: Psychotic syndromes in epilepsy. Am J Psychiatry 142:895–904, 1985

McNeil TF: Obstetric factors and perinatal injuries, in Handbook of Schizophrenia, Vol 3: Nosology, Epidemiology and Genetics of Schizophrenia. Edited by Tsuang MT, Simpson FC. New York, Elsevier, 1988

McNeil TF, Kaij L: Obstetric factors in the development of schizophrenia: complications in the birth of preschizophrenics and in reproduction by schizophrenic parents, in The Nature of Schizophrenia. Edited by Wynne LC, Cromwell RL, Matthysee S. New York, John Wiley, 1978, pp 401–429

Mednick SA, Machon RA, Huttunen MO, et al: Adult schizophrenia following prenatal exposure to an influenza epidemic. Arch Gen Psychiatry 45:189–192, 1988

Meehl PE: Schizotaxia, schizotypy, schizophrenia. Am J Psychiatry 17:827–838, 1962

Meltzer HY: Biology of schizophrenia subtypes: a review and proposal for method study. Schizophr Bull 5:460–479, 1979

Meltzer HY: Dopamine and negative symptoms in schizophrenia: critique of type I-type II hypothesis, in Controversies in Schizophrenia: Changes and Consistencies. Edited by Alpert M. New York, Guilford, 1984, pp 110–144

Meltzer HY: Neuroendocrinology of schizophrenia, in Neuroendocrinology and Psychiatric Disorder. Edited by Brown GM, Koslow SH, Reichlin S. New York, Raven, 1985, pp 1–28

Meltzer HY: Biological studies of the nosology of the major psychoses: a status report on the schizoaffective disorders, in Schizoaffective Psychoses. Edited by Maneros A, Tsuang MT. Berlin, Springer-Verlag, 1986, pp 232–259

Meltzer HY: Biological studies in schizophrenia. Schizophr Bull 13:77–111, 1987

Meltzer HY: Clinical studies on the mechanism of action of clozapine: the dopamine-serotonin hypothesis of schizophrenia. Psychopharmacology 99 (Suppl):518–527, 1989

Meltzer HY: Negative symptoms in schizophrenia: a target of new drug development, in Clinical Pharmacology in Psychiatry, Vol 3. Edited by Dahl SG, Gram LF. Berlin, Springer-Verlag (in press)

Meltzer HY, Busch DA: Serum prolactin response to chlorpromazine and psychopathology in schizophrenics: implications for the dopamine hypothesis. Psychiatry Res 9:285, 1983

Meltzer HY, Busch DA: Serum prolactin response to chlorpromazine and psychopathology in schizophrenia. Psychiatr Clin North Am 9:99–113, 1986

Meltzer HY, Stahl SM: The dopamine hypothesis of schizophrenia: a review. Schizophr Bull 2:19–76, 1976

Meltzer HY, Kolakowska T, Fang VS, et al: Growth hormone and prolactin response to apomorphine in schizophrenia and the major affective disorders. Arch Gen Psychiatry 41:512–519, 1984

Meltzer HY, Sommers AA, Luchins DJ: The effect of neuroleptics and other psychotropic drugs on negative symptoms in schizophrenia. J Clin Psychopharmacol 6:329–338, 1986

Meltzer HY, Bastani B, Ramirez LF, et al: Clozapine: new research on efficacy and mechanism of action. Eur Arch Psychiatry Neurol Sci 238:332–339, 1989a

Meltzer HY, Bastani B, Kwon KY: A prospective study of clozapine in treatment-resistant schizophrenic patients, I: preliminary Report. Psychopharmacology 99 (suppl):568–572, 1989b

Merriam AE, Kay SR, Opler LA, et al: Neurological signs and the positive-negative dimension in schizophrenia. Biol Psychiatry 28:181–192, 1990

Mielke DH, Gallant DM, Roniger JJ, et al: Sulpiride: evaluation of anti-psychotic activity in schizophrenic patients. Diseases of the Nervous System 38:569–571, 1977

Milner B: Some effects of frontal lobectomy in man, in The Frontal Granular Cortex and Behavior. Edited by Warren JM, Akert K. New York, McGraw-Hill, 1963, pp 313–334

Modestin J, Schwartz RB, Hunger J: Zur frage der beeinflussung schizophrener symptome durch physostigmin. Pharmakopsychiatr Neuropsychopharmakol 9:300–304, 1973

Moller HJ, Kissling W, Bottermann P: The dexamethasone suppression test in depressive and schizophrenic patients under controlled conditions. Eur Arch Psychiatry Neurol Sci 235:263–268, 1986

Morley JE: Neuroendocrine control of thyrotrophin secretion. Endocr Rev 2:396–436, 1981

Morley MJ, Shah K, Bradshaw CM, et al: DSP4 and Hernstein's equation: further evidence for a role of noradrenaline in the maintenance of operant behavior by positive reinforcement. Psychopharmacology (Berlin) 96:551–556, 1988

Morrison RL, Bellack AS, Mueser KT: Deficits in facial-affect recognition and schizophrenia. Schizophr Bull 14:67–83, 1988

Moscarelli M, Maffei C, Cesana BM, Boato P, Farma T, Grilli A, Lingiardi V, Cazzullo CL: An international perspective on assessment of negative and positive symptoms in schizophrenia. Am J Psychiatry 144:1595–1598, 1987

Mosher LR, Meltzer HY: Neuroleptics and psychosocial treatment. Schizophr Bull 6:8–9, 1980

Muller-Spahn F, Ackenheil M, Albus M, et al: Neuroendocrine effects of apomorphine in chronic schizophrenic patients under long-term neuroleptic therapy and after drug withdrawal: relationship to psychopathology and tardive dyskinesia. Psychopharmacology (Berlin) 84:436–440, 1984

Muller-Spahn F, Ackenheil M, Albus M: Neuroendocrine effects of clonidine in chronic schizophrenic patients under long-term neuroleptic therapy and after drug withdrawal: relations to psychopathology. Psychopharmacology (Berlin) 88:190, 1986

Murphy MR, MacLean PD, Hamilton SC: Species-typical behavior of hamsters deprived from birth of the neocortex. Science 213:459–461, 1981

Murray RM, Lewis SW: Is schizophrenia a neurodevelopmental disorder? (editorial). Br Med J 295:681–682, 1987

Murray RM, Lewis SW, Reveley AM: Towards an aetiological classification of schizophrenia. Lancet 1:1023–1026, 1985

Murray RM, Reveley AM, McGuffin P: Genetic vulnerability to schizophrenia. Psychiatr Clin North Am 9:3–16, 1986

Murray RM, Lewis SW, Owen MJ, et al: The neurodevelopmental origins of dementia praecox, in Schizophrenia: The Major Issue. Edited by Bebbington P, McGuffin P. London, Heinemann Professional Publishing, 1988, pp 90–106

Myers RE, Swett C: Social behavior deficits of free-ranging monkeys after anterior temporal cortex removal: a preliminary report. Brain Res 18:551–556, 1970

Myers RE, Swett C, Miller M: Loss of social group affinity following prefrontal lesions in free-ranging macaques. Brain Res 64:257–269, 1973

Naber D, Albus M, Burke H, et al: Neuroleptic withdrawal in chronic schizophrenia: clinical and endocrine variables relating to psychopathology. Psychiatry Res 16:207–219, 1985

Nasrallah HA, Wilcox JA: Gender differences in the etiology and symptoms of schizophrenia: genetic versus brain injury factors. Annals of Clinical Psychiatry 1:51–53, 1989

Nasrallah HA, McCalley Whitters M, Jacoby CG: Cortical atrophy in schizophrenia and mania: a comparative CT study. J Clin Psychiatry 43:439–441, 1982

Nasrallah HA, Kuperman S, Jacoby CG, et al: Clinical correlates of sulcal widening in chronic schizophrenia. Psychiatry Res 10:237–242, 1983a

Nasrallah HA, Kuperman S, Hamra BJ, et al: Clinical differences between schizophrenic patients with and without large cerebral ventricles. J Clin Psychiatry 44:407–409, 1983b

National Institute of Mental Health, Psychopharmacology Service Center Collaborative Study Group: Phenothiazine treatment in acute schizophrenia. Arch Gen Psychiatry 10:246–261, 1964

National Institute of Mental Health, Psychopharmacology Service Center Collaborative Study Group: Clinical effects of three phenothiazines in acute schizophrenia. Diseases of the Nervous System 28:369–383, 1967

Nauta WJH: The problem of the frontal lobe: a reinterpretation. J Psychiatr Res 8:167–187, 1971

Nyback H, Berggren B, Hindmarsh T, et al: Cerebroventricular size and cerebrospinal fluid monoamine metabolites in schizophrenic patients and healthy volunteers. Psychiatry Res 9:301–308, 1983

Obiols JE, Salvador L, Humbert M, et al: Evalucion de las sintomas negativos de la esquizofrenia. Rev Depart Psiq Fac Med Barcelona 12:85–91, 1985

Obiols JE, Marcos JE, Salamero M: Ventricular enlargement and neuro-psychological testing in schizophrenia. Acta Psychiatr Scand 76:199–202, 1987

Opler LA, Kay SR, Rosado V, et al: Positive and negative syndromes in chronic schizophrenic inpatients. J Nerv Ment Dis 172:317–325, 1984

Opler LA, Kay SR, Fiszbein A: Positive and negative syndromes in schizophrenia: typological, dimensional, and pharmacological validation, in Positive and Negative Symptoms in Psychosis: Description, Research, and Future Directions. Edited by Harvey PD, Walker E. Hillsdale, NJ, Lawrence Erlbaum, 1987, pp 124–154

Ornstein K, Milon H, McRae-Degueurce A, et al: Biochemical and radioautographic evidence for dopaminergic afferents of the locus coeruleus originating in the ventral tegmental area. J Neural Transm 70:183–191, 1987

O'Rourke DH, Gottesman II, Suarez BK, et al: Refutation of the general single locus model in the aetiology of schizophrenia. Am J Hum Genet 34:630–649, 1982

Overall JE: The Brief Psychiatric Rating Scale in psychopharmacology research, in Psychological Measurements in Psychopharmacology, Modern Problems in Pharmacopsychiatry, Vol 7. Edited by Pichot P. Basel, Karger, 1974, pp 67–78

Overall JE, Gorham DR: Brief Psychiatric Rating Scale. Psychol Rep 10:799–812, 1962

Overall JE, Rhodes JV: Refinement of phenomenological classification in clinical psychopharmacology research. Psychopharmacology 77:24–30, 1982

Overall JE, Hollister LE, Pichot P: A four dimensional model. Arch Gen Psychiatry 9:280–294, 1963

Owen F, Cross AJ, Crow TJ, et al: Increased dopamine receptor sensitivity in schizophrenia. Lancet 2:223–226, 1978

Owen F, Crow TJ, Frith CD, et al: Selective decreases in MAO-B activity in postmortem brains from schizophrenic patients with the type II syndrome. Br J Psychiatry 151:514–519, 1987

Owen MJ, Lewis SW, Murray RM: Family history and cerebral ventricular enlargement in schizophrenia: a case control study. Br J Psychiatry 154:629–634, 1989a

Owen MJ, Lewis SW, Murray RM: Obstetric complications and schizophrenia: a computed tomographic study. Psychol Med 18: 332–340, 1989b

Owens DGC, Johnstone EC: The disabilities of chronic schizophrenia: their nature and the factors contributing to their development. Br J Psychiatry 136:384–395, 1980

Owens DGC, Johnstone EC, Frith CD: Spontaneous involuntary disorders of movement. Arch Gen Psychiatry 39:452–461, 1982

Owens DGC, Johnstone EC, Crow TJ, et al: Lateral ventricular size in schizophrenia: relationship to the disease process and its clinical manifestations. Psychol Med 15:27–41, 1985

Pandey GN, Garver DL, Tamminga C, et al: Postsynaptic supersensitivity in schizophrenia. Am J Psychiatry 134:518–522, 1977

Pandurangi AK, Dewan MJ, Boucher M, et al: A comprehensive study of chronic schizophrenic patients, II: biological, neuropsychological, and clinical correlates of CT abnormality. Acta Psychiatr Scand 73:161–171, 1986

Pandurangi AK, Bilder RM, Rieder RO, et al: Schizophrenic symptoms and deterioration: relation to computed tomography findings. J Nerv Ment Dis 176:200–206, 1988

Pandurangi AK, Goldberg SC, Brink DD, et al: Amphetamine challenge test, response to treatment, and lateral ventricle size in schizophrenia. Biol Psychiatry 25:207–214, 1989

Parnas J, Schulsinger F, Schulsinger H, et al: Behavioral precursors of schizophrenia spectrum: schizophrenia. Psychiatr Clin North Am 9:99–103, 1986

Pearlson GD, Garbacz DJ, Breakey WR, et al: Lateral ventricular enlargement associated with persistent unemployment and negative symptoms in both schizophrenia and bipolar disorder. Psychiatry Res 12:1–9, 1984

Pearlson GD, Garbacz DJ, Moberg PJ, et al: Symptomatic, familial, perinatal, and social correlates of computed axial tomography (CAT) changes in schizophrenics and bipolars. J Nerv Ment Dis 173:42–50, 1985

Penfield W, Evans J: The frontal lobe in man: a clinical study of maximum removals. Brain 58:115–133, 1935

Pepeu G, Bartolini A: Effect of psychoactive drugs on the output of acetylcholine from the cerebral cortex of the cat. Eur J Pharmacol 4:254–263, 1968

Perez MM, Trimble MR: Epileptic psychosis: diagnostic comparison with process schizophrenia. Br J Psychiatry 137:245–249, 1980

Peselow E, Angrist B, Sudilovsky A, et al: Double blind controlled trials of cholecystokinin octapeptide in neuroleptic-refractory schizophrenia. Psychopharmacology 91:80–84, 1987

Petho B, Bitter I: Types of complaints in psychiatric and internal medical patients. Psychopathology 18:241–253, 1985

Pfeiffer CC, Jenney EH: The inhibition of conditional response and counteraction of schizophrenia by muscarinic stimulation of the brain. Ann NY Acad Sci 66:753–764, 1957

Phillips L: Case history data and prognosis in schizophrenia. J Nerv Ment Dis 117:515–525, 1953

Pickar D, Breier A, Hsiao JK, et al: Cerebrospinal and plasma monoamine metabolites and their relation to psychosis. Arch Gen Psychiatry 47:641–648, 1990

Ploog D: Neurobiology of primate audio-vocal behavior. Brain Res Rev 3:35–61, 1981

Pogue-Geile MF: Longitudinal characteristics of negative symptoms in schizophrenia. Br J Psychiatry 155 (Suppl 7):123–127, 1989

Pogue-Geile MF, Harrow M: Negative and positive symptoms in schizophrenia and depression: a follow-up. Schizophr Bull 10:371–387, 1984

Pogue-Geile MF, Harrow M: Negative symptoms in schizophrenia: their longitudinal course and prognostic importance. Schizophr Bull 11:427–439, 1985

Pogue-Geile MF, Harrow M: Negative symptoms, affective deficit states, and intellectual dysfunction in chronic schizophrenia, in Anhedonia and Affect Deficit States. Edited by Clark D, Fawcett J. New York, SP Medical & Scientific Books, 1987a

Pogue-Geile MF, Harrow M: Negative symptoms in schizophrenia: longitudinal characteristics and etiological hypotheses, in Positive and Negative Symptoms in Psychosis: Description, Research, and Future Directions. Edited by Harvey PD, Walker E. Hillsdale, NJ, Lawrence Erlbaum, 1987b, pp 94–123

Pogue-Geile MF, Hogarty G: Phenotypic differences among schizophrenic patients: their association with familial risk for schizophrenia. Abstracts of the second annual meeting of the Society for Research on Psychopathology, Atlanta. Atlanta, GA, Society for Research on Psychopathology, 1987

Pogue-Geile MF, Zubin J: Negative symptomatology in schizophrenia: a conceptual and empirical review. International Journal of Mental Health 16:3–45, 1988

Poplawsky A, Johnson DA: Open-field social behavior of rats following lateral or medial septal lesions. Physiol Behav 11:845–854, 1973

Popper KR: Conjectures and Reflections. London, Routledge & Kegan Paul, 1963

Post RM, Fink E, Carpenter WT Jr, et al: Cerebrospinal fluid amine metabolites in acute schizophrenia. Arch Gen Psychiatry 32:1063–1069, 1975

Powchik P, Davis BM, Davis KL: The neuroendocrinology of schizophrenia, in Handbook of Schizophrenia, Vol 2: Neurochemistry and Neuropharmacology. Edited by Henn FA, DeLisi LE. New York, Elsevier, 1987, pp 337–376

Prange AJ, Loosen PT, Wilson IC, et al: Behavioral and endocrine response of schizophrenic patients to TRH (protirelin). Arch Gen Psychiatry 36:1086–1093, 1979

Prien RF: Problems and practices in geriatric psychopharmacology. Psychosomatics 21:213–223, 1980

Prien RF, Cole JO: High dose chlorpromazine therapy in chronic schizophrenia. Arch Gen Psychiatry 18:482–495, 1968

Prien RF, Levine J, Cole JO: High dose trifluoperazine therapy in chronic schizophrenia. Am J Psychiatry 126:305–313, 1969

Purves D, Lichtman JW: Principles of Neural Development. Sunderland, MA, Sinauer Associates, 1985

Pycock CJ, Kerwin RW, Carter CJ: Effect of lesion of cortical dopamine terminals on subcortical dopamine in rats. Nature 286:74–77, 1980

Rado S: Psychoanalysis of Behavior. New York, Grune & Stratton, 1956

Rakic P, Bourgeois JP, Eckenhoff MF, et al: Concurrent overproduction of synapses in diverse regions of the primate cerebral cortex. Science 232:232–235, 1986

Randrup A, Munkvad I: Special antagonism of amphetamine-induced abnormal behavior: inhibition of stereotyped activity with increase in some normal activities. Psychopharmacologia 7:416–422, 1965

Rasmussen DD, Liu JH, Wolf PL, et al: Gonadotropin releasing hormone secretion in the human hypothalamus: in vitro regulation by dopamine. J Clin Endocrinol Metab 62:479–483, 1986

Raz N, Raz S, Bigler ED: Ventriculomegaly in schizophrenia: the role of control groups and the perils of dichotomous thinking. Psychiatry Res 26:245–248, 1988

Reich T, James JW, Morris CA: The use of multiple thresholds in determining the mode of transmission of semicontinuous traits. Ann Hum Genet 36:163–183, 1972

Reitan RM: Halstead-Reitan Neuropsychological Test Battery. Tucson, AZ, Neuropsychology Laboratory, University of Arizona, 1979

Reveley MA, Reveley AM, Baldy R: Left hemisphere hypodensity in discordant schizophrenic twins: a controlled study. Arch Gen Psychiatry 44:625–632, 1987

Richelson E: Neuroleptic affinities for human brain receptors and their use in predicting adverse effects. J Clin Psychiatry 45:331–336, 1984

Rifkin A, Quitkin F, Klein DF: Akinesia: a poorly recognized drug-induced extrapyramidal behavioral disorder. Arch Gen Psychiatry 32:672–674, 1975

Risch SC, Cohen RM, Janowsky DS, et al: Physostigmine induction of depressive symptomatology in normal human subjects. Psychiatry Res 4:89–94, 1981

Roberts GW, Ferrier IN, Lee Y, et al: Peptides, the limbic lobe and schizophrenia. Brain Res 288:199–211, 1983

Roberts GW, Colter N, Lofthouse R, et al: Gliosis in schizophrenia: a survey. Biol Psychiatry 21:1043–1050, 1986

Roberts GW, Colter N, Lofthouse R, et al: Is there gliosis in schizophrenia? Investigation of the temporal lobe. Biol Psychiatry 22:1459–1468, 1987

Robinson SE: Cholinergic pathways in the brain, in Central Cholinergic Mechanisms and Adaptive Dysfunctions. Edited by Singh MM, Warburton DM, Lal H. New York, Plenum, 1985, pp 37–61

Rogers D: The motor disorders of severe psychiatric illness: a conflict of paradigms. Br J Psychiatry 147:221–232, 1985

Rosen WG, Mohs RC, Johns CA, et al: Positive and negative symptoms in schizophrenia. Psychiatry Res 13:277–284, 1984

Rosenthal R, Bigelow LB: The effects of physostigmine in phenothiazine resistant chronic schizophrenic patients. Compr Psychiatry 14:489–494, 1973

Rossi A, de Cataldo S, Stratta P, et al: Cerebral atrophy and neuropsychological correlates in schizophrenia. Acta Psychiatr Belg 87:670–675, 1987

Rosvold HE, Mirsky AF, Pribram KH: Influence of amygdalectomy on social behavior in monkeys. Journal of Comparative and Physiological Psychology 47:173–178, 1954

Roth S: The seemingly ubiquitous depression following acute schizophrenic episodes. Am J Psychiatry 127:91–98, 1970

Rotrosen J, Angrist BM, Gershon S: Dopamine receptor alteration in schizophrenia: endocrine evidence. Psychopharmacology 51:1–122, 1976

Rotrosen J, Angrist B, Clark C, et al: Suppression of prolactin by dopamine agonists in schizophrenics and normal controls. Am J Psychiatry 135:949–951, 1979

Rowntree DW, Nevin S, Wilson A: The effects of disopropylfluorophosphate in schizophrenia and manic-depressive psychosis. J Neurol Neurosurg Psychiatry 13:47–62, 1950

Rutter M: Epidemiological approaches to developmental psychopathology. Arch Gen Psychiatry 45:486–495, 1988

Saffer D, Metcalfe M, Coppen A: Abnormal dexamethasone suppression test in Type II schizophrenia? Br J Psychiatry 147:721–723, 1985

Scatton B, Rouquier L, Javoy-Agid F, et al: Dopamine deficiency in the cerebral cortex in Parkinson disease. Neurology 32:1039–1040, 1982

Scharfetter C: Subdividing the functional psychoses: a family hereditary approach. Psychol Med 11:637–640, 1981

Scheinin M, Chang W-H, Kirk JL, et al: Simultaneous determination of 3-methoxy-4 hydroxyphenylglycol 5-hydroxyindolacetic acid, and homovanillic acid in CSF with high performance liquid chromatography using electrochemical detection. Anal Biochem 131:246–253, 1983

Schimmelbusch WH, Muller PS, Sheps J: Insulin resistance and duration of hospitalization in untreated schizophrenics. Br J Psychiatry 118:429–436, 1971

Schizophrenia Bulletin: Issue theme: Negative symptoms in schizophrenia. Volume II, Whole Issue 3

Schneider K: Clinical Psychopathology. Translated by Hamilton MW. New York, Grune & Stratton, 1959

Scoville WB, Dunsmore RH, Liberson WT, et al: Observations on medical temporal lobotomy and uncotomy in the treatment of psychotic states. Proc Assoc Res Nerv Ment Dis 31:347–369, 1953

Sedvall G, Alfredsson G, Bjerkenstedt L, et al: Central biochemical correlates to antipsychotic drug action in man, in The Impact of Biology on Modern Psychiatry. Edited by Gerson ES, Belmaker RH, Kety SS, et al. New York, Plenum, 1976, pp 41–54

Seeman P, Lee T: Antipsychotic drugs: direct correlation between clinical potency and presynaptic action on dopamine neurons. Science 188:1217–1219, 1975

Seeman P, Lee T, Chau-Wong M, et al: Antipsychotic drug doses and neuroleptic/dopamine receptors. Nature 261:717–719, 1976

Serafetinides EA, Collins S, Clark MI: Haloperidol, clopenthixol and chlorpromazine in chronic schizophrenia. J Nerv Ment Dis 154:31–42, 1972

Shelton RC, Weinberger DR: X-ray computerized tomography studies in schizophrenia: a review and synthesis, in The Neurology of Schizophrenia, Vol 1. Edited by Nasrallah HA, Weinberger DR. Amsterdam, Elsevier, 1986, pp 207–250

Shelton RC, Karson CN, Doran AR, et al: Cerebral structural pathology in schizophrenia: evidence for a prefrontal cortical deficit. Am J Psychiatry 145:154–163, 1988

Sheppard GP: High dose propranolol in schizophrenia. Br J Psychiatry 134:470–476, 1979

Sherrington R, Brynjolfsson J, Petursson H, et al: Localisation of a susceptibility locus for schizophrenia on chromosome 5. Nature 336:164–167, 1988

Singh MM, Kay SR: A comparative study of haloperidol and chlorpromazine in terms of clinical effects and therapeutic reversal with benztropine in schizophrenia: theoretical implications for potency differences among neuroleptics. Psychopharmacologia 43:103–113, 1975a

Singh MM, Kay SR: A longitudinal therapeutic comparison between two prototypic neuroleptics (haloperidol and chlorpromazine) in matched groups of schizophrenics: nontherapeutic interactions with trihexyphenidyl; theoretical implications for potency differences. Psychopharmacologia 43:115–123, 1975b

Singh MM, Kay SR: Wheat gluten as a pathogenic factor in schizophrenia. Science 191:401–402, 1976

Singh MM, Kay SR: Dysphoric response to neuroleptic treatment in schizophrenia: its relationship to autonomic arousal and prognosis. Biol Psychiatry 14:277–294, 1979a

Singh MM, Kay SR: Therapeutic antagonism between anti-parkinsonism medication and neuroleptics in schizophrenia: implications for a neuropharmacological model. Neuropsychobiology 5:74–86, 1979b

Singh MM, Kay SR: Pharmacology of central cholinergic mechanisms and schizophrenic disorders, in Central Cholinergic Mechanisms and Adaptive Functions. Edited by Singh MM, Warburton DM, Lal H. New York, Plenum, 1985, pp 247–308

Singh MM, Kay SR: Is the positive-negative distinction in schizophrenia valid? Br J Psychiatry 150:879–880, 1987

Singh MM, Lal H: Central cholinergic mechanisms, neuroleptic action, and schizophrenia, in Clinical Applications of Neuropharmacology. Edited by Essman WB, Valzelli L. New York, Spectrum, 1982, pp 337–389

Singh MM, Smith JM: Sleeplessness in acute and chronic schizophrenia: response to haloperidol and anti-parkinsonism agents. Psychopharmacologia 29:21–32, 1973

Singh MM, Kay SR, Opler LA: Anticholinergic-neuroleptic antagonism in terms of positive and negative symptoms of schizophrenia: implications for psychobiological typing. Psychol Med 17:39–48, 1987

Siris SG, van Kammen DP, Docherty JP: Use of antidepressants in schizophrenia. Arch Gen Psychiatry 35:1368–1377, 1978

Siris SG, Morgan V, Fagerstrom R, et al: Adjunctive imipramine in the treatment of postpsychotic depression. Arch Gen Psychiatry 44:533–539, 1987

Sitaram N, Moore AM, Gillin JC: Scopolamine-induced muscarinic super-sensitivity in normal man: changes in sleep. Psychiatry Res 1:9–16, 1979

Slater E, Roth M: Clinical Psychiatry, 3rd Edition. Baltimore, MD, Williams & Wilkins, 1969

Slater E, Beard AW, Clithero E: The schizophrenia-like psychoses of epilepsy. Br J Psychiatry 109:95–150, 1963

Smith GN, Iacono WG: Ventricular size in schizophrenia: importance of choice of control subjects. Psychiatry Res 26:241–243, 1988

Smith JM: Abuse of the antiparkinson drugs: a review of the literature. J Clin Psychiatry 41:351–354, 1980

Smith RC, Baumgartner R, Ravichandran GK, et al: Lateral ventricular enlargement and clinical response in schizophrenia. Psychiatry Res 14:241–253, 1984

Snezhnevsky AV: The symptomatology, clinical forms and nosology of schizophrenia, in Modern Perspectives in World Psychiatry. Edited by Howells JG. Edinburgh, Oliver & Boyd, 1968, pp 425–447

Snyder S, Greenberg D, Yamamura HI: Antischizophrenic drugs and brain cholinergic receptors. Arch Gen Psychiatry 31:58–61, 1974

Sommers AA: "Negative symptoms": conceptual and methodological problems. Schizophr Bull 11:364–379, 1985

Sorokin JE, Giordani B, Mohs RC, et al: Memory impairment in schizophrenic patients with tardive dyskinesia. Biol Psychiatry 23:129–135, 1988

Spitzer RL, Endicott J, Robins E: Research Diagnostic Criteria: rationale and reliability. Arch Gen Psychiatry 35:773–782, 1978

Spitzer R, Williams J, Gibbon M: Structured Clinical Interview for DSM-III-R. New York, Biometrics Research Department, New York State Psychiatric Institute, 1986

Stahl SM, Uhr SB, Berger PA: Pilot study on the effects of fenfluramine on negative symptoms in twelve schizophrenic inpatients. Biol Psychiatry 20:1098–1102, 1985

Stahl SM, Jernigan T, Pfefferbaum A, et al: Brain computerized tomography in subtypes of severe chronic schizophrenia. Psychol Med 18:73–77, 1988

Stanley M, Traskman-Bendz L, Dorovini-Zio K: Correlations between aminergic metabolites simultaneously obtained from human CSF and brain. Life Sci 37:1279–1286, 1985

Stein L, Wise CD: Possible etiology of schizophrenia: progressive damage to the noradrenergic reward system by 5-hydroxydopamine. Science 171:1032–1036, 1971

Steklis HD, Kling AJ, Ervin F: The influence of selective ablations of the temporal lobe on social behavior of the vervet. J Med Primatol 4:357–358, 1975

Sternberg DE, van Kammen DP, Lake CP, et al: The effect of pimozide on CSF norepinephrine in schizophrenia. Am J Psychiatry 138:1045–1051, 1981

Sternberg DE, van Kammen DP, Lerner P, et al: Schizophrenia: dopamine-beta-hydroxylase activity and treatment response. Science 216:1423–1425, 1982

Sternberg DE, van Kammen DP, Lerner P, et al: CSF dopamine beta-hydroxylase in schizophrenia. Arch Gen Psychiatry 40:743–747, 1983

Strauss JS, Carpenter WT: The prediction of outcome in schizophrenia. Arch Gen Psychiatry 27:739–746, 1972

Strauss JS, Carpenter WT: The Psychiatric Assessment Interview (PAI). New Haven, CT, Yale University, 1974

Strauss JS, Carpenter WT, Bartko JJ: The diagnosis and understanding of schizophrenia, part 3: speculations on the processes that underlie schizophrenic symptoms and signs. Schizophr Bull 11:61–75, 1974

Strauss JS, Klorman R, Kokes RF: Premorbid adjustment in schizophrenia: concepts, measures, and implications, V: the implications of findings for understanding, research, and application. Schizophr Bull 3:240–244, 1977

Stuss DT, Benson DF: The Frontal Lobes. New York, Raven, 1986

Szechtman H, Nahmias C, Garnett ES, et al: Effect of neuroleptics on altered cerebral glucose metabolism in schizophrenia. Arch Gen Psychiatry 45:523–532, 1988

Takahashi R, Inanaga V, Kato N, et al: CT scanning and the investigation of schizophrenia, in Biological Psychiatry. Edited by Perris C, Struwe G, Jansson B. Amsterdam, Elsevier, 1982, pp 259–268

Tamminga CA, Smith RC, Pandey G, et al: A neuroendocrine study of supersensitivity in tardive dyskinesia. Arch Gen Psychiatry 34:1199–1203, 1977

Tandon R, Greden JF: Cholinergic hyperactivity and negative schizophrenic symptoms: a model of dopaminergic/cholinergic interactions in schizophrenia. Arch Gen Psychiatry 46:745–753, 1989

Tandon R, Greden JF, Silk KR: Treatment of negative schizophrenic symptoms with trihexiphenidyl. J Clin Psychopharmacol 8:212–215, 1988

Tandon R, Shipley J, Eiser A, et al: Association between abnormal rapid eye movement sleep and negative symptoms in schizophrenia. Psychiatry Res 27:359–361, 1989a

Tandon R, Mazzara C, Silk KR: DST in schizophrenia: reply to Keshavan et al. Biol Psychiatry 26:858, 1989b

Tandon R, Shipley J, DeQuardo J, et al: EEG sleep abnormalities in schizophrenia: relationship to positive/negative symptoms and ventricular size. Biol Psychiatry 25:180–181, 1989c

Tandon R, Goodson J, Silk KR, et al: Positive and negative symptoms in schizophrenia and the dexamethasone suppression test. Biol Psychiatry 25:788–792, 1989d

Tandon R, Mann NA, Eisner WE, et al: Effect of anticholinergic medication on positive and negative symptoms in medication-free schizophrenic patients. Psychiatry Res 31:235–241, 1990a

Tandon R, Goldman RS, Goodson J, et al: Mutability and relationship between positive and negative symptoms during neuroleptic treatment in schizophrenia. Biol Psychiatry 27:1323–1326, 1990b

Tandon R, DeQuardo J, Goldman R, et al: Psychotic-phasic and deficit-enduring subtypes of negative symptoms: Biological markers and relationship to outcome. Biol Psychiatry 27:101–102A, 1990c

Tandon R, Shipley JE, Greden JF, et al: Muscarinic cholinergic hyperactivity in schizophrenia: relationship to positive and negative symptoms. Schizophrenia Research (in press a)

Tandon R, Mazzara C, DeQuardo J, et al: Dexamethasone suppression test in schizophrenia: relationship to symptomatology, ventricular enlargement, and outcome. Br J Psychiatry (in press b)

Targum SD: Neuroendocrine dysfunction in schizophreniform disorder: correlation with six months outcome. Am J Psychiatry 140:309–313, 1983

Taylor MA, Abrams R: A rating scale for emotional blunting. Am J Psychiatry 135:226–229, 1978

Terzian H, Ore GD: Syndrome of Kluver and Bucy reproduced in man by bilateral removal of the temporal lobes. Neurology 5:373–380, 1955

Thaker G, Buchanan RW, Kirkpatrick B, et al: Eye movements in schizophrenia: clinical and neurobiological correlates. Abstracts Society of Neuroscience 14:339, 1988

Thiemann S, Csernansky JG, Berger PA: Rating scales in research: the case of negative symptoms. Psychiatry Res 20:47–55, 1987

Thierry A-M, Tassin JP, Glowinski J: Biochemical and electrophysical studies of the mesocortical dopamine system, in Monoamine Innervation of Cerebral Cortex. Edited by Descarsies L, Reader TR, Jasper HH. New York, Alan R Liss, 1984, pp 233–262

Toone BK, Garralda ME, Ron MA: The psychosis of epilepsy and the functional psychoses: a clinical and phenomenological comparison. Br J Psychiatry 141:256–261, 1982

Torgerson S: Relationship of schizotypal personality disorder to schizophrenia: genetics. Schizophr Bull 11:554–563, 1985

Toru M, Moriya H, Yamamoto K, et al: A double-blind comparison of sulpiride with chlorpromazine in chronic schizophrenia. J Clin Pharmacol 12:221–229, 1972

Toumisto J, Mannisto P: Neurotransmitter regulation of anterior pituitary hormones. Pharmacol Rev 37:249–332, 1985

Trimble MR: First-rank symptoms of Schneider: a new perspective? Br J Psychiatry 156:195–200, 1990

Tsuang MT, Winokur GW: Criteria for subtyping schizophrenia: clinical differentiation of hebephrenic and paranoid schizophrenia. Arch Gen Psychiatry 31:43–47, 1974

Uematsu M, Kaiya H: The morphology of the corpus callosum in schizophrenia: a MRI study. Schizophrenia Research 1:391–398, 1988

van Kammen DP, Antelman SM: Impaired noradrenergic transmission in schizophrenia? A minireview. Life Sci 34:1403–1413, 1984

van Kammen DP, Boronow JJ: Dextro-amphetamine diminishes negative symptoms in schizophrenia. Int Clin Psychopharmacol 3:111–121, 1988

van Kammen DP, Gelernter J: Biochemical instability in schizophrenia, I: the norepinephrine system, in Psychopharmacology: The Third Generation of Progress. Edited by Meltzer HY. New York, Raven, 1987, pp 745–751

van Kammen DP, Malas KL, Sternberg DE, et al: Platelet MAO and clinical variables in schizophrenia: interrelationships with spinal fluid NE and DBH. Psychopharmacol Bull 17:207–209, 1981

van Kammen DP, Docherty JP, Bunney WE: Prediction of early relapse after pimozide discontinuation by response to d-amphetamine during pimozide treatment. Biol Psychiatry 17:233–242, 1982

van Kammen DP, Mann LS, Sternberg DE, et al: Dopamine beta-hydroxylase activity and homovanillic acid in spinal fluid of schizophrenic patients with brain atrophy. Science 220:974–976, 1983

van Kammen DP, Rosen J, Peters J, et al: Are there state-dependent markers in schizophrenia? Psychopharmacol Bull 21:497–502, 1985a

van Kammen DP, Mann LS, Scheinin M, et al: Decreased spinal fluid monoamine metabolites and norepinephrine in schizophrenic patients with brain atrophy, in Pathochemical Markers in Major Psychoses. Edited by Beckmann H, Reiderer P. New York, Springer-Verlag, 1985b, pp 88–95

van Kammen DP, van Kammen WB, Peters JL, et al: CSF MHPG, sleep and psychosis in schizophrenia. Clin Neuropharmacol 9:575–577, 1986a

van Kammen DP, van Kammen WB, Mann LS, et al: Dopamine metabolism in the cerebrospinal fluid of drug-free schizophrenic patients with and without cortical atrophy. Arch Gen Psychiatry 43:978–983, 1986b

van Kammen DP, Hommer DW, Malas KL: Effect of pimozide on positive and negative symptoms in schizophrenic patients: are negative symptoms state dependent? Neuropsychobiology 18:113–117, 1987

van Kammen DP, van Kammen WB, Peters J, et al: Decreased slow-wave sleep and enlarged lateral ventricles in schizophrenia. Neuropsychopharmacology 1:265–271, 1988

van Kammen DP, Peters J, van Kammen WB, et al: CSF norepinephrine in schizophrenia is elevated prior to relapse after haloperidol withdrawal. Biol Psychiatry 26:176–188, 1989

van Kammen DP, Peters J, Yao J, et al: Norepinephrine in acute exacerbations of chronic schizophrenia: negative symptoms revisited. Arch Gen Psychiatry 47:161–168, 1990

van Putten T, Mutalipassi LR, Malkin MD: Phenothiazine-induced decompensation. Arch Gen Psychiatry 30:102–105, 1974

Vance MA, Blumberg JB: Cholinergic potentiation of neuroleptic effects in the nucleus accumbens. Res Commun Chem Pathol Pharmacol 40:345–348, 1983

Vaughn M, Krawiecka M: Sensitivity to change in symptoms of new scales for rating chronic psychotic patients. International Pharmacopsychiatry 14:121–126, 1977

Vieweg WVR, David JJ, Rowe WT, et al: Psychogenic polydipsia and water intoxication: concepts that have failed. Biol Psychiatry 20:1308–1320, 1985

Vigneri R, Pezzino V, Sqatrito S, et al: Sleep-associated growth hormone release in schizophrenia. Neuroendocrinology 14:356, 1974

Vita A, Sachetti E, Calzeroni A, et al: Cortical atrophy in schizophrenia: prevalence and associated features. Schizophrenia Research 1:329–337, 1988

Volkow ND, Wolf AP, Van Gelder P, et al: Phenomenological correlates of metabolic activity in 18 patients with chronic schizophrenia. Am J Psychiatry 144:151–158, 1987

Waddington JL, Crow TJ: Abnormal involuntary movements in the pre-neuroleptic era and in unmedicated patients: implications for the concept of tardive dyskinesia, in Tardive Dyskinesia: Biological Mechanisms and Clinical Aspects. Edited by Wolf ME, Mosnaim A. Washington, DC, American Psychiatric Press, 1988, pp 49–66

Wagman AMI, Heinrichs DW, Carpenter WT: The deficit and non-deficit forms of schizophrenia: neuropsychological evaluation. Psychiatry Res 22:319–330, 1987

Waldhauser F, Weiszenbacher G, Frisch H, et al: Fall in nocturnal serum melatonin during prepuberty and pubescence. Lancet 1:362–365, 1984

Walker EF: Validating and conceptualizing positive and negative symptoms, in Positive and Negative Symptoms of Psychosis. Edited by Harvey PD, Walker EF. Hillsdale, NJ, Lawrence Erlbaum, 1987, pp 30–49

Walker E, Lewine RRJ: The positive/negative symptom distinction in schizophrenia: validity and etiological relevance. Schizophrenia Research 1:315–328, 1988

Walker E, Harvey PD, Perlman D: The positive/negative symptom distinction in psychoses: a replication and extension of previous findings. J Nerv Ment Dis 176:359–363, 1988

Wallace CJ, Liberman RP: Social skills training for patients with schizophrenia: a controlled clinical trial. Psychiatry Res 15:239–247, 1985

Watt NF, Grubb TW, Erlenmeyer-Kimling L: Social, emotional, and intellectual behavior at school among children at high risk for schizophrenia, in Children at High Risk for Schizophrenia: A Longitudinal Perspective. Edited by Watt NF, Anthony EJ, Wynne LC, et al. New York, Cambridge University Press, 1984, pp 171–181

Wechsler D: Wechsler Adult Intelligence Scale–Revised. San Antonio, TX, Psychological Corporation, 1981

Weinberger DR: Implications of normal brain development for the pathogenesis of schizophrenia. Arch Gen Psychiatry 44:660–669, 1987

Weinberger DR, Torrey EF, Andreas NN, et al: Lateral cerebral ventricular enlargement in chronic schizophrenia. Arch Gen Psychiatry 36:735–739, 1979

Weinberger DR, Bigelow LB, Kleinman JE, et al: Cerebral ventricular enlargement in chronic schizophrenia: association with poor response to treatment. Arch Gen Psychiatry 37:11–14, 1980a

Weinberger DR, Cannon-Spoor E, Potkin SG, et al: Poor premorbid adjustment and CT scan abnormalities in chronic schizophrenia. Am J Psychiatry 137:1410–1413, 1980b

Weinberger DR, Berman KF, Zec RF: Physiological dysfunction of dorsolateral prefrontal cortex in schizophrenia, I: regional cerebral blood flow (rCBF) evidence. Arch Gen Psychiatry 43:114–125, 1986

Weinberger DR, Berman KF, Chase TN: Mesocortical dopaminergic function and human cognition. Ann NY Acad Sci 537:330–338, 1988a

Weinberger DR, Berman KF, Illowsky BP: Physiological dysfunction of dorsolateral prefrontal cortex in schizophrenia, III: a new cohort and evidence for a monoaminergic mechanism. Arch Gen Psychiatry 45:609–615, 1988b

Whalley LJ, Christie JE, Brown S, et al: Schneider's first rank symptoms of schizophrenia: an association with increased growth hormone response to apomorphine. Arch Gen Psychiatry 41:1040–1043, 1984

Wik G, Wiesel F-A, Eneroth P, et al: Dexamethasone suppression test in schizophrenic patients before and during neuroleptic treatment. Acta Psychiatr Scand 74:161–167, 1986

Williams AO, Reveley MA, Kolakowska T, et al: Schizophrenia with good and poor outcome, II: cerebral ventricular size and its clinical significance. Br J Psychiatry 146:239–246, 1985

Wing JK: A simple and reliable subclassification of chronic schizophrenia. Journal of Mental Science 107: 862–875, 1961

Wing JK, Brown GW: Institutionalism and Schizophrenia. New York, Cambridge University Press, 1970

Wing JK, Brown GW: Institutionalism and schizophrenia, in Schizophrenia: Towards a New Synthesis. Edited by Wing JK. London, Academic, 1978

Wing JK, Cooper JE, Sartorius N: Measurement and Classification of Psychiatric Symptoms: An Instruction Manual for the PSE and Catego Program. New York, Cambridge University Press, 1974

Wise RA: Neuroleptics and operant behavior: the anhedonia hypothesis. Behavioral and Brain Sciences 5:39–87, 1982

Withers E, Hinton J: Three forms of the clinical tests of the sensorium and their reliability. Br J Psychiatry 119:1–8, 1971

Woggon B, Angst M, Bartels K, et al: Antipsychotic efficacy of fluperlapine. Neuropsychobiology 18:113–117, 1984

Wolkin A, Peselow ED, Smith M, et al: TRH test abnormalities in psychiatric disorders. J Affective Disord 6:273–281, 1984

Wolkowitz OM, Pickar D, Doran AR, et al: Combination alprazolam-neuroleptic treatment of the positive and negative symptoms of schizophrenia. Am J Psychiatry 143: 85–87, 1986

Wolkowitz OM, Breier A, Doran A, et al: Alprazolam augmentation of the antipsychotic effects of fluphenazine in schizophrenic patients. Arch Gen Psychiatry 45:664–671, 1988

Wong DF, Wagner HN, Tune LE, et al: Positron emission tomography reveals elevated D_2 dopamine receptors in drug-naive schizophrenics. Science 234:1558–1560, 1986

World Health Organization: Report of the International Pilot Study of Schizophrenia, Vol 1. Geneva, Switzerland, World Health Organization Press, 1974

Yarbrough GG: On the neuropharmacology of thyrotropin releasing hormone. Prog Neurobiol 12:291–312, 1979

Yaryura-Tobias JA, Wolpert A, Dand L, et al: Action of L-dopa in drug-induced extrapyramidalism. Diseases of the Nervous System 31:60–63, 1970a

Yaryura-Tobias JA, Diamond B, Merlis S: The action of L-dopa on schizophrenic patients (a preliminary report). Current Therapeutic Research 12:528–531, 1970b

Zagrodzka J, Brudnias-Stepowska Z, Fonberg E: Impairment of social behavior in amygdalar cats. Acta Neurobiol Exp (Warsz) 43:114–125, 1983

Zarcone VP, Benson KL, Berger PA: Abnormal rapid eye movement latencies in schizophrenia. Arch Gen Psychiatry 44:45–48, 1987

Zatz LM, Jernigan TL: The ventricular-brain ratio on computed tomography scans: validity and proper use. Psychiatry Res 8:207–214, 1983

Zemlan FP, Hirschowitz J, Garver DL: Relation of clinical symptoms to apomorphine-stimulated growth hormone release in mood-incongruent psychotic patients. Arch Gen Psychiatry 43:1162–1167, 1986a

Zemlan FP, Hirschowitz J, Sautter F, et al: Relationship of psychotic symptom clusters in schizophrenia to neuroleptic treatment and growth hormone response to apomorphine. Psychiatry Res 18:239–255, 1986b

Zubin J: Negative symptoms: are they indigenous to schizophrenia? Schizophr Bull 11:461–470, 1985